WE BELIEVE
FOOD IS MEDICINE

WE BELIEVE IN
KINDNESS TO ALL ALL SPECIES

WE BELIEVE
IN A SUSTAINABLE ENVIRONMENT

WE BELIEVE
LIFE MUST BE COLORFUL

WE BELIEVE IN
ORGANICALLY AWESOME FOOD

The material in this book is for informational purposes only and is not intended as a substitute for the advice and care of your physician. As with all new diet and nutrition regimens, the program described in this book should be followed only after first consulting with your physician to make sure it is appropriate to your individual circumstances. The author and publisher expressly disclaim responsibility for any adverse effects that may result from the use or application of the information contained in this book.

Copyright © 2021 by Nastasha McKeon

All rights reserved.

Nastasha@choicejuicery.com

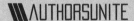

Published by Authorsunite.com

Names: McKeon, Nastasha, author.
Title: Plant Food Is Medicine
Subjects: Over 100 Organic, Plant-Based and Gluten-Free Recipes from Choice Juicery

Printed in the United States of America

Cover and book design by: Michael Gonsalves (Zeachman Design)
Photographs by: Kerry Kaestner, Hannah Towery, Robby Gogatz
Editors: Kathalyn Nakashima, Harshini Wijesuriya, Sheree Trask and Michael Gonsalves

Second Edition

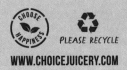

WWW.CHOICEJUICERY.COM

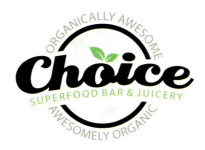

ACKNOWLEDGEMENT

I want to thank my kids for their love, support and presence in my life, which has always inspired me to strive to do my best to leave this world a better place than I found it. Thank you Mikey, Tessa and Kora for always inspiring me to be more. I want to thank my Choice family for making Choice and this book possible. Especially Kathalyn Nakashima (Naka!). I want to thank Tom Penn for teaching me so much, and for encouraging me to write this book. I want to thank Patrick Farley for believing in me before I believed in myself and for giving me confidence in my healthy creations. I would like to thank my Grandma Lola for her presence in my life, even though she left this planet too soon. Losing her ultimately inspired my journey into health and wellness, which lead to Choice and this book becoming a reality. I want to thank my mom for overcoming all that she has, becoming a huge presence in my life and for helping so much with my kiddos, which has allowed me to do what I do with Choice and the creation of this book. I want to thank my brothers for all of their support and encouragement throughout this journey. And last but not least, I want to thank my Choice designer Michael Gonsalves, my photographer Kerry Kaestener and my editors for making the MAGIC in these pages come together.

YOU CANNOT GET THROUGH A SINGLE DAY WITHOUT HAVING AN IMPACT ON THE WORLD AROUND YOU. WHAT YOU DO MAKES A DIFFERENCE, AND YOU HAVE TO DECIDE WHAT KIND OF DIFFERENCE YOU WANT TO MAKE.

-Jane Goodall

Every time you sit down to eat, you are making a choice that will impact this planet, and our food choices can help or harm this beautiful world. Making food choices that are more sustainable for our planet makes a huge difference. When people tell me that they don't think what they do really matters (although there are billions of people on this planet), I am reminded of one of my favorite stories, "The Boy and the Starfish".

Once upon a time, there was an old man who liked to go to the ocean to write. He made it a practice to walk on the beach every morning before he began his work. Early one day, while he walked along the shore after a big storm had passed, he found the vast beach littered with starfish as far as the eye could see, stretching in both directions.

Off in the distance, the old man noticed a small boy approaching. The man watched the boy walk along the beach. As he grew closer, the man could see the boy bend down every so often, to pick up an object and throw it into the sea. The boy came closer still and the man called out, "Good morning! May I ask what it is that you are doing?"

The young boy paused, looked up, and said, "Throwing starfish into the ocean. The tide has washed them up onto the beach and they can't return to the sea by themselves. When the sun gets high, they will die, unless I throw them back into the water."

The old man replied, "But there must be tens of thousands of starfish on this beach. I'm afraid you won't really be able to make much of a difference."

The boy bent down, picked up yet another starfish and threw it as far as he could into the ocean. Then he turned, smiled and said, "It made a difference to that one!"

Adapted from <u>The Star Thrower</u>, *by Loren Eiseley (1907 – 1977)*

CONTENTS

INTRODUCTION 10

CHAPTER ONE
PLANT POWER
14

CHAPTER TWO
WHY JUICE?
24

CHAPTER THREE
JUICES
34

CHAPTER FOUR
PLANT-BASED MILKS
44

CHAPTER FIVE
ELIXIRS & LATTÉS
54

CHAPTER SIX
SUPERFOOD SMOOTHIES
72

CHAPTER SEVEN
SMOOTHIE BOWLS
90

CHAPTER EIGHT
WRAPS
100

CHAPTER NINE
SUSHI
118

CHAPTER TEN
SALADS
136

CHAPTER ELEVEN
SOUPS
146

CHAPTER TWELVE
NOODLES
156

CHAPTER THIRTEEN
SNACKS
166

CHAPTER FOURTEEN
SWEET TREATS
172

CHAPTER FIFTEEN
SAUCES, DRESSINGS & TOPPINGS
188

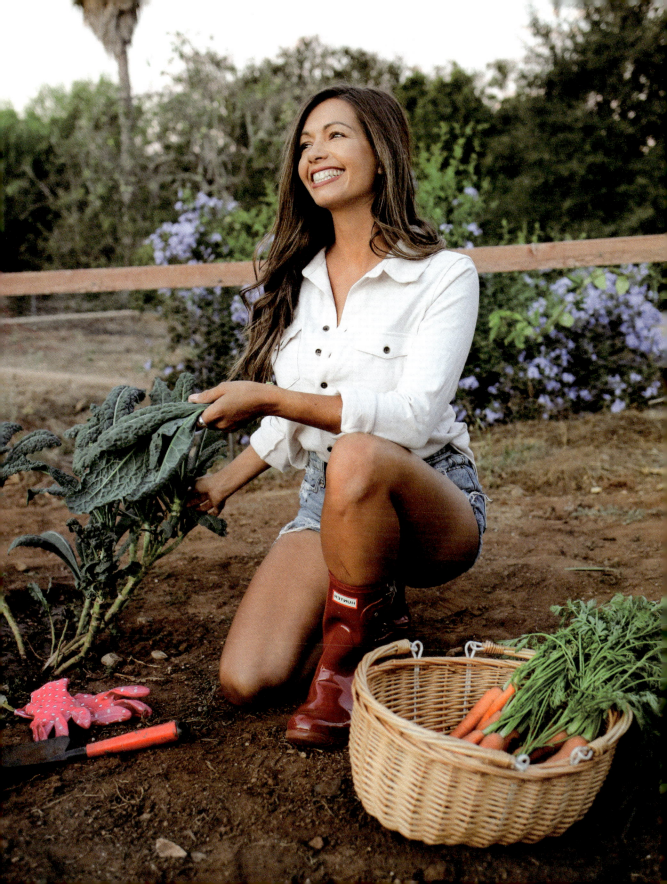

INTRODUCTION

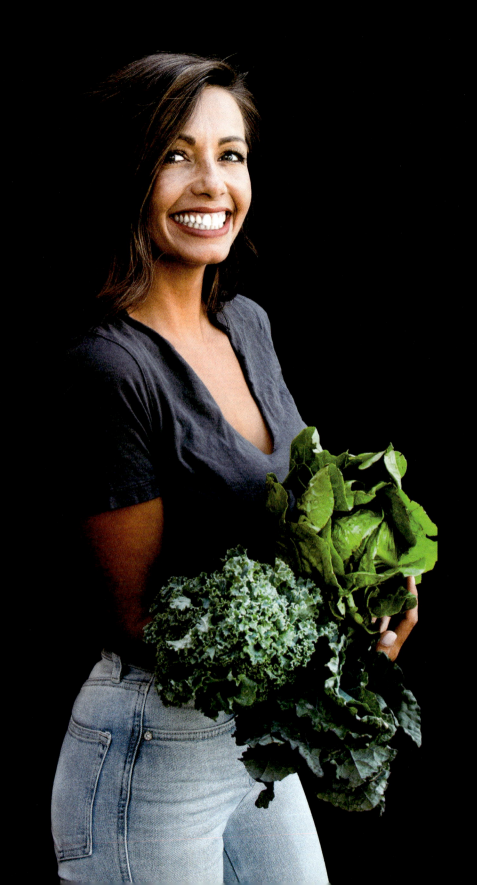

Hi

I'm Nastasha McKeon, the founder of Choice Superfood Bar and Juicery. You may have seen me bouncing around the stores— sometimes with a few kiddos in tow— as I'm usually at several of our locations each and every day.

This recipe book has been a labor of love and I'm so excited to finally share it with you. Health and wellness is my greatest passion in life, which is why I created a juicery and superfood bar (and this book!) - to make quality nutrition not only delicious, but accessible. I get so much joy out of sharing awesome, organic food with the incredible communities we are blessed to serve. I wanted to take my passion and our company mission of sharing healthy food to the next level by bringing you into my kitchen, and sharing some of my favorite recipes with you in hopes of inspiring you further on your path to living a happy, healthy, and holistically-minded lifestyle.

Before we dive into all of this yumminess, I would like to share a little bit about my personal journey that ultimately led to the creation of Choice, and the book in your hands right now. My desire to do so stems from really wanting people to understand the power of food, and our ability to heal - no matter your circumstances.

Like many others, my upbringing was a bit rocky. The road to get to where I am today has not been easy, but I can say with 100% certainty that it has absolutely been worth it! I grew up in a severely abusive environment, experiencing and seeing things that I'd never wish upon another human. On top of that, food was scarce and I found myself in a constant state of fight or flight. As I grew up, I realized that simply being a part of the human experience meant that pain (to some degree) was inevitable - but suffering was a choice.

One of the most pivotal moments for me happened when I was 11 years old, and I lost my grandma to an autoimmune disease. She was everything to me! Losing someone close to you at any age is tough, but for me, having it happen at such a young age was a tragedy on a massive scale. She was my only light in a very dark childhood, and taken away from me far too soon. My grandmother was diagnosed with scleroderma and within a year she went from a strong, active and vibrant woman to a frail, sick human reliant on an oxygen tank for air. It was devastating to watch and confusing to understand.

While I knew she was ill, her death felt rather sudden. She ultimately died from complications of a prescription drug she was given to treat the symptoms of her disease.

A week after my grandmother's passing, I was at her house helping to clear out her belongings. It was then that I stumbled upon a book in her room that she never had the chance to read. The book was all about the idea that *food was medicine*, a concept that I'd never been exposed to previously. I remember picking it up and being intrigued. As I read through the pages, I found myself immediately hooked! The book went on to discuss the power of our food choices in disease prevention - and even treatment. This was so foreign to me, but it spoke to a part of me that I didn't even know existed. In that moment, my passion and love for nutrition, health and wellness was born. Although the seed had been planted, I did not have the right circumstances to help me cultivate this newfound passion until a bit later in life, but the nagging in my soul was loud and persistent and eventually, it became impossible to ignore.

Turning Passion Into Purpose

Fast forward many years later, I was now an adult managing life as a single mom with a solid career in the banking industry. Although by many people's standards I was doing really well, there was still something missing and no matter what I did, nothing seemed to fill the void.

I found myself going through the motions of life, unfulfilled and constantly searching for deeper meaning. I'll never forget the day that one of my banking customers came in and told me something that completely changed my life. *"Nastasha, if you love what you do, you'll never work another day in your life."*

While a common saying, it was the first time I'd heard it and it struck a chord with me. What had I been doing all these years? This couldn't possibly be all there was to life! So instead of wondering, and wishing things would change, I made it my mission to figure out what exactly it was that I loved doing, outside of being a mom. And come to find out, all that I'd been searching for was found in the breakroom.

I hadn't really paid much attention up to that point, but looking back, people were always curious about what I was eating - and I loved to share! I loved talking about food, and exposing others to the benefits of making healthy choices. And more than anything, I loved bringing extra food into the bank breakroom for anyone that wanted to try something new. I also secretly loved the idea of shattering the belief that healthy food had to taste terrible! In fact, nothing was more rewarding for me.

Over the years, I watched so many people experience major changes in their health due to our conversations, and it lit me up. I watched people reverse diabetes and get off insulin. I watched people lose weight and become more active. Right before my eyes I was witnessing people's mental health improve because of the quality nutrition they were putting into their bodies. When I realized how powerful even a simple conversation could be, and what was possible when people chose better for themselves and their families, there was no turning back. I knew that I wanted to continue inspiring people to make better choices, which meant going to school to study nutrition. Soon after this realization, I left banking and began teaching plant-based cooking and nutrition classes all over San Diego, CA. I was in heaven!

Just like so many others with a passion burning hot in their belly, there was a moment along the way that solidified everything I'd been working so hard for.

I was teaching a class at Scripps Medical Center as a part of their Employee Wellness Program. I had been teaching there for several months and I felt like I was really making a difference. Week after week, people were reaping the benefits of the food I was sharing, while learning how they could make the recipes on their own at home. They always left so inspired, only to return the following day overwhelmed by the fact that actually putting these recipes together at home felt "too hard."

And it dawned on me...

I knew that simply showing people how to make healthy food that actually tasted good wasn't enough, it needed to be convenient too. That was my aha moment, and the day I knew that I wanted to create a place that did just that. Sure there were restaurants that had healthy options on the menu, but it's hard to make good choices when you've got the smell of french fries hitting you in the face the moment you arrive. I wanted to open a place where making a "bad" choice wasn't even an option because everything on the menu was not only incredibly nourishing, but so good that people would crave coming back for more.

And that is how Choice Superfood Bar and Juicery was born.

The Choice is Yours

One of the first things you'll notice when you visit Choice Juicery, aside from our positive vibes and happy energy, are the messages written on our walls and printed on our shirts. "Choose Happiness" and "Be Kind" aren't just company mottos, they are the core values we choose to operate from. Choice gives both myself, and my team, the opportunity to share love and kindness with our communities, spread happiness with all those we come in contact with, and share the knowledge that Plant Food is Medicine.

It's been an incredible journey with lots of ups and downs. But no matter what comes my way, I wake up in gratitude each and every day for having the opportunity to serve my community using healthy, organic food choices that are in alignment with my nutritional philosophy. At Choice, we are so proud and honored to do what we love, and what we believe in. Through every item purchased, we're making a positive impact on the health of our community, and our environment, which is really what it's all about. And sharing the recipes in this book makes our mission and movement that much sweeter (without all the added sugar).

It brings me so much joy to do my part to empower you to make delicious Choice foods in the comfort of your own home. Organic, vegan & gluten-free. Everything within these pages was created with you in mind.

Thank you so much for all of your continued support. We couldn't do it without you.

NASTASHA MCKEON

Nastasha McKeon

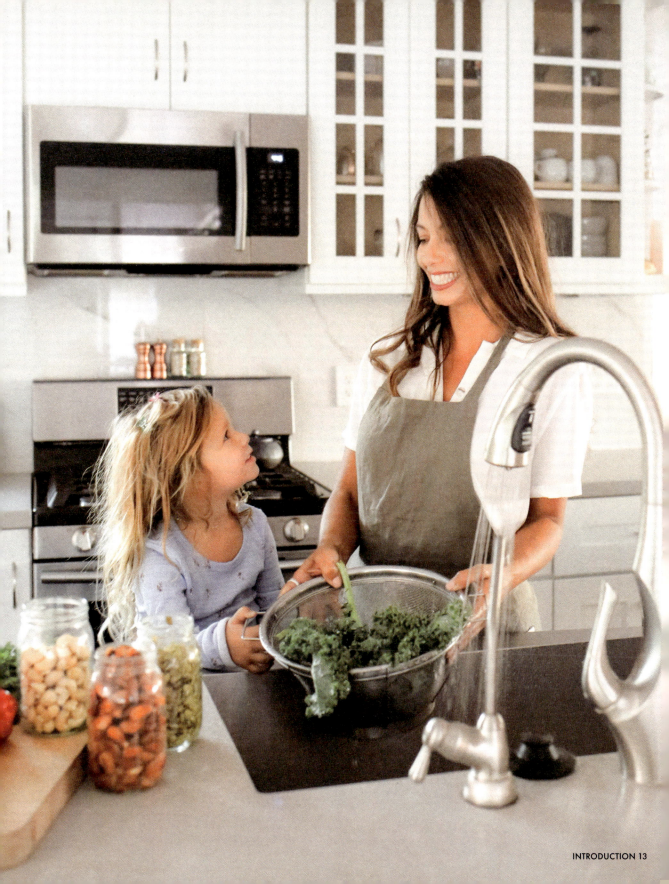

CHAPTER 1

WHY *Plant*-BASED?

FOR THE PLANET, FOR YOUR HEALTH & FOR THE ANIMALS

I get this question a lot and it's actually one of my favorite questions to answer. But before I dive into it, I want to say that I am an advocate for progress over perfection. I believe the great majority of us are genuinely trying to do the best we can with what we know. I celebrate that. I celebrate every plant-based choice made and I'm thankful for every single bit of forward progress.

When it comes to my nutritional philosophy, it's pretty simple and it boils down to three main factors.

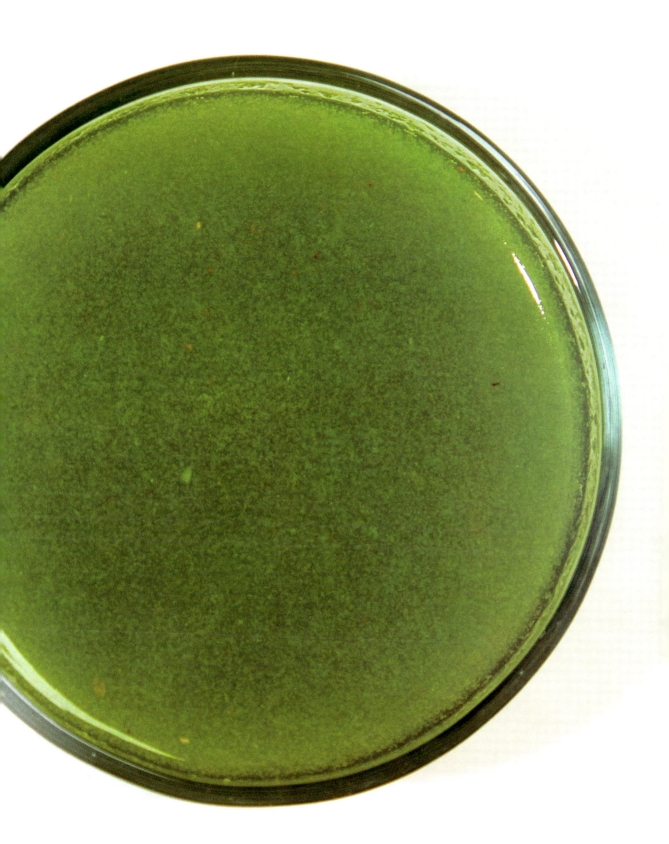

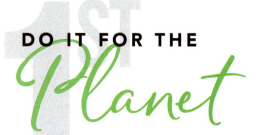

DO IT FOR THE *Planet*

Ditching meat and dairy is the most impactful step an individual can take to lessen their impact on the planet. We aren't just talking greenhouse gases, but global acidification, eutrophication, land use and water use. It is far bigger than cutting down on your flights, buying an electric car, or using energy efficient lightbulbs. The science is unanimous: the best change we can each make to help our planet is to stop eating animal products.

Here are some statistics that you may or may not be familiar with:

- Each day, a person who eats a vegan diet saves 1,100 gallons of water, 45 pounds of grain, 30 sq ft of forested land, 20 lbs carbon dioxide (CO_2) equivalent, and one animal's life.

- A person who follows a vegan diet produces the equivalent of 50% less carbon dioxide, uses 1/11th the oil, 1/13th the water, and 1/18th the land compared to a meat-lover for their food.

- 30% of the world's total ice-free surface — is used not to raise grains, fruits and vegetables that are directly fed to human beings, but to support the chickens, pigs and cattle that we eventually eat.

- Livestock covers 45% of the Earth's total land.

- Cows produce 150 billion gallons of methane per day.

- Livestock operations on land have created more than 500 nitrogen flooded dead zones around the world in our oceans.

- Hog, chicken and cattle waste has polluted 35,000 miles of rivers in 22 states and contaminated groundwater in 17 states.

- Growing feed crops for livestock consumes 56% of the water supply in the U.S.

- We are in the midst of the largest mass extinction in 65 million years.

- Nearly half of the contiguous U.S. is devoted to animal agriculture.

- 33% of the planet is desertified, with livestock as the leading driver.

- Animal agriculture is responsible for 20%-33% of all freshwater consumption in the world today.

- 2,500 gallons of water are needed to produce 1 pound of beef.

- Livestock and their byproducts account for at least 32 million tons of CO_2 per year, or 51% of all worldwide greenhouse gas emissions.

- Livestock is responsible for 65% of all human-related emissions of nitrous oxide – a greenhouse gas with 296 times the global warming potential of carbon dioxide CO_2, and which stays in the atmosphere for 150 years.

- A farm with 2,500 dairy cows produces the same amount of waste as a city of 411,000 people.

- Animal agriculture is the leading cause of species extinction, ocean dead zones, water pollution, and habitat destruction.

- 75% of the world's fisheries are exploited or depleted.

- We could see fishless oceans by 2048.

- 90-100 million tons of fish are pulled from our oceans each year.

- As many as 2.7 trillion animals are pulled from the ocean each year.

- Animal agriculture is responsible for the destruction of up to 91% of the Amazon rainforest.

- 1-2 acres of rainforest are cleared every second.

- The leading causes of rainforest destruction are livestock and feed crops.

- Up to 137 plant, animal and insect species are lost every day due to rainforest destruction.

- 136 million rainforest acres have been cleared for animal agriculture.

- 1,100 land activists have been killed in Brazil in the past 20 years.

- Ten thousand years ago, 99% of biomass (i.e. zoomass) was wild animals. Today, humans and the animals that we raise as food make up 98% of the zoomass.

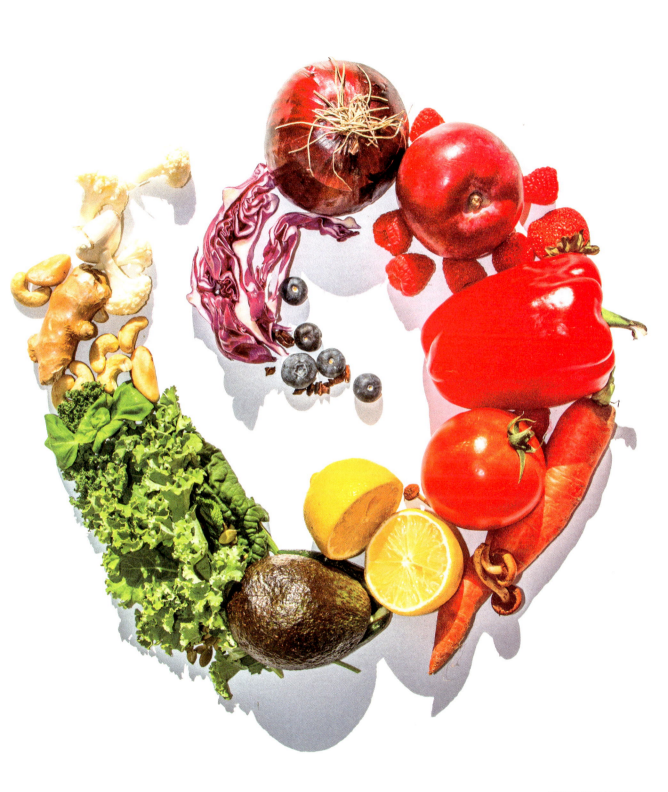

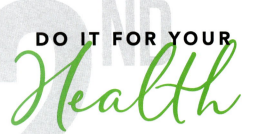

DO IT FOR YOUR Health

A whole foods vegan diet can be one of the healthiest ways to live. It may contribute to a higher daily intake of fruits, vegetables, whole grains, beans, legumes, nuts and seeds. Because vegan diets often rely heavily on these healthy staples, they tend to be higher in vitamins, minerals, antioxidants, phytochemicals, and fiber. They are also richer in potassium, magnesium, folic acid, iron and vitamins A, C, B1 and E while also being significantly lower in cholesterol and saturated fats.

A vegan diet based around nutrient-rich whole plant foods may reduce the risk of developing type 2 diabetes, cardiovascular disease, hypertension, stroke, obesity and some cancers including; prostate, breast, and colon cancers. A vegan diet can be healthy for anyone of any age, including children, the elderly, pregnant and nursing women.

Here are a few facts about animal products and the potential health impacts:

- World Health Organization reports have classified bacon & sausage as carcinogenic to humans.

- One serving of processed meat per day increases the risk of developing diabetes by 51%.

- Eating 1 egg per day is just as bad as smoking 5 cigarettes per day for life expectancy.

- The number one source of saturated fat is dairy.

- The egg industry funds studies that confuse consumers.

- The strategy of the meat, dairy & egg industry is to confuse the public, to introduce doubt not unlike the tobacco industry.

- Concerns regarding consuming fish include: pcb's, mercury, saturated fat and cholesterol.

- Fish have become mercury sponges.

- Toxins bioaccumulate in fish flesh.

- Commercial animals are largely fed genetically modified (GMO) corn and soy.

- Eating organic meat will not help you avoid contaminants.

- Most of the world's GMO crops are consumed by livestock with dairy cows consuming the most per animal.

- There is a strong link between dairy foods and autoimmune diseases.

- Most people in the world are lactose intolerant.

- Milk is a hormonal fluid.

- Milk does not build strong bones—countries with the highest rates of dairy consumption have the highest rates of osteoporosis.

- Dairy is linked to many different types of cancer.

- Any animal protein boosts the level of cancer promoting growth hormone igf-1.

- Dairy products increase the risk of cancers related to your hormones.

- Dairy can increase a man's risk of getting prostate cancer by 34%.

- For women who have had breast cancer, just one serving of whole dairy a day can increase their chances of dying from the disease by 49%, and dying from any disease by 64%.

- Casein protein, the main protein in dairy products, especially in cheese, creates casomorphins—casomorphin may play a role in sudden infant death syndrome (SIDS) and autism.

- There are at least 450 animal drugs, drug combinations, and other feed additives that are administered to animals to achieve increased growth and keep them alive in conditions that would otherwise kill them.

- Pharmaceutical industry sells 80% of all antibiotics made in the United States to animal agriculture.

- 3,000 People die each year in the United States from food borne illnesses.

- 23,000 People die each year from antibiotic-resistant bacteria.

- The World Health Organization said that we are nearing a post-antibiotic era in medicine.

- Dead hogs are processed into feed and fed back to the hogs.

- A low fat, plant-based diet is more than twice as powerful at controlling and/or reversing diabetes, than the American Diabetes Association (ADA) diet recommending meat and dairy.

- Studies reference a link between exposure to dairy at a young age and type 1 diabetes.

- Cow milk protein causes antibodies in the bloodstream that attack the pancreas.

- USDA dietary committee members have received money from animal products, sugar and alcohol industries.

- USDA admitted that eggs cannot legally be labeled: nutritious, low fat, part of a balanced diet, low calorie, healthful, healthy, good for you, or safe.

- The dairy industry spends at least $50 million promoting its products in public schools.

- The meat and dairy industry spends at least $138 million lobbying congress.

- In the U.S, treating chronic disease is a $1.5 trillion industry.

- The American Cancer Society, American Diabetes Association and American Heart Association have accepted millions of dollars from pharmaceutical companies.

- Testing shows 88% of pork chops, 90% of ground beef and 95% of chicken breasts sampled were contaminated with fecal bacteria.

> **All protein is initially made by plants**

- Plants are loaded with protein.

- Most Americans get about twice the protein they need.

- Most Americans get less than half of the fiber they need.

- Human milk has the lowest protein content of any other species.

- The largest, strongest terrestrial animals on the planet are all herbivores.

- Humans closest living relatives are chimpanzees, who get 97% of their calories from plants.

- You can stop and reverse heart disease with plant-based diets.

- When people adopt a fully plant-based diet, their cholesterol levels plummet within a few days.

- When people adopt a fully plant-based diet, blood pressure comes down.

> **99.4% Were able to avoid major cardiac events by going plant-based**

- Crohn's disease & multiple sclerosis remission rates are best achieved from a plant-based diet.

- The power of food is not taught in medical school.

- The Academy of Nutrition and Dietetics puts out nutrition fact sheets from the industries themselves.

- If you eat meat, the chances of getting diabetes are about 1 in 3.

- If you eat meat, the chances of getting cancer if you're a man are 1 in 2, if you're a woman 1 in 3.

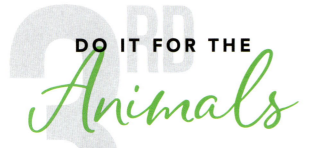

DO IT FOR THE Animals

Many people identify themselves as animal lovers, yet intentionally (or unintentionally), this doesn't always extend to the animals we use for food. Before going vegan, this was me. There are a lot of misconceptions about how animal products are obtained and we often turn a blind eye towards inhumane animal agricultural practices. Animal welfare is an issue I pushed out of my mind for years. Ignorance was bliss. I learned the power of association, or rather disassociation, in my early 20's.

I had disassociated the meat on my plate with the animals that it had come from. It was easier to turn a blind eye than to seriously question how these foods ended up on my plate and into my body. One day, I was watching the news during a huge mad cow disease meat recall, and was exposed to what a factory farm looked like. As I sat watching in horror, the camera zeroed in on cows (very much alive and very much in pain) as they were being moved into a discard pile with a fork lift. They were being treated like a commodity (which unfortunately today, they are), instead of the living, breathing, feeling sentient beings that they are. For a moment, the camera paused on a cow that was being moved as she moaned in agony. I saw her eyes, and I could feel the fear, pain and confusion. For the first time, I felt empathy for what I had always looked at as "just food" and it broke me.

I learned early on as a child (as most of us do) not to look, feel and or care about the animals we eat because we are so conditioned to believe that we must eat these "things" in order to be healthy. But on that particular day, everything I had once believed changed and I never ate a cow again. I started to see meat for what it was: dead animals that likely endured a lot of pain and suffering before being slaughtered to satisfy my taste buds. It wasn't long after that I learned about all of the animal abuse involved with animal products, which I had been eating my whole life. As I learned more, I continued to change my nutritional philosophy until eventually, I was completely vegan.

Factory farming exhibits some of the most severe examples of animal cruelty for food production. Unfortunately, factory farming offers the most competitive prices and makes the most profit, so it's difficult and in some cases, impossible for smaller establishments to survive without adopting the same practices. Factory farming is an absolutely horrifying business, with a focus on production and profit, instead of the well-being of the animals and workers involved. It all comes down to money.

Here are some facts on animal agriculture:

- 70 Billion farmed animals are reared annually worldwide. More than 6 million animals are killed for food every hour.

- A battery chicken lives on space smaller than your iPad. They have no room to turn around, and certainly not enough space to stretch their wings. They also have to spend their entire lives standing on metal mesh flooring, which causes pain, discomfort, and injury to the feet and legs.

- Animals are forced to grow up to three times faster than nature intended.

- Due to selective breeding and the use of weight gaining drugs in feed, animals are forced to grow at an alarming rate.

- Dairy cows are killed after just three lactation cycles. The natural lifespan of a cow is between 20 to 25 years. However, in factory farms, dairy cows are often considered to be "spent" by the time they have gone through just three lactation cycles. They are aggressively bred, fed, and drugged to produce as much milk as possible in the shortest amount of time, and this has a detrimental effect on their overall health and long term milk production. In the modern farming world, it's more cost effective to send them to the slaughter at this early stage of life and have them replaced before their milk production decreases.

- Newborn animals are routinely mutilated. Piglets are mutilated within the first two weeks of life by having their teeth clipped, tails cut off, and testicles removed. This is done without anesthetic, and is incredibly painful to the animals. It is done to prevent the pigs from damaging themselves and each other when they become agitated and distressed due to their cramped living conditions. Chickens have their beaks clipped for the same reason.

- Mothers are separated from their babies at birth. In the dairy industry, calves are taken away from their mothers at birth and are sent off to veal farms where they will spend the rest of their short lives. The calves are not allowed to stay with their mothers as they would drink their mother's milk, which is desired by the industry for human consumption instead. In the pork industry, piglets are weaned from their mothers after just two weeks so that the sow can be made pregnant again, as this increases the amount of litters she can produce each year.

- An incredible 99% of farmed animals are now bred in factory farms. This means that due to current accepted regulations on animal welfare in these farms, 99% of farmed animals in the U.S. will never get to exhibit their natural behaviors. Pigs love to bathe in the sun, snuffle in the mud, and create complex social relationships, yet in factory farms, they are confined to tiny pens for their entire lives. Chickens love to flap their wings and clean themselves in dust baths, yet the cages they are confined to prevent them from standing up straight, or even stretching their wings. Cows enjoy grazing in fields, yet are also confined to concrete pens where the range of movement is limited to sitting or standing.

- 2 in 3 farm animals in the world are now factory farmed.

- Egg-laying hens are sometimes starved for up to 14 days, exposed to changing light patterns and given no water in order to shock their bodies into molting. It's common for 5% to 10% of hens to die during the forced molting process.

- As much as 40% (63 billion pounds) of fish caught globally every year are discarded.

- For every 1 pound of fish caught, up to 5 pounds of unintended marine species are caught and discarded as by-kill.

- Scientists estimate as many as 650,000 whales, dolphins and seals are killed every year by fishing vessels.

> **Ag-Gag Laws criminalize whistle-blowers who photo-document abuses by the animal agriculture industry**

For more information or for fact sources, please visit the following:

www.whatthehealthfilm.com/facts
www.cowspiracy.com
www.dosomething.org/us/facts/11-facts-about-animals-and-factory-farms
www.onegreenplanet.org/animalsandnature/facts-about-the-lives-of-factory-farmed-animals/
www.dosomething.org/us/facts/11-facts-about-animals-and-factory-farms

If you are interested in learning more about this topic in general, here are a few documentaries I highly recommend:

- Cowspiracy (Netflix)
- What the Health (Netflix)
- Speciesism (Netflix)
- Forks Over Knives (Netflix)
- Earthlings (Youtube)
- Meet your Meat (Youtube)

Books:
- Eating Animals
- The China Study
- The Food Revolution
- Diet For A New America
- The Cheese Trap

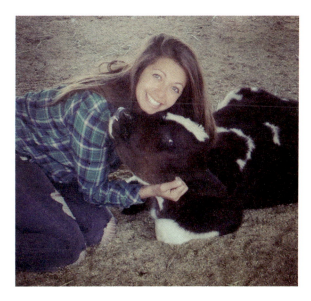

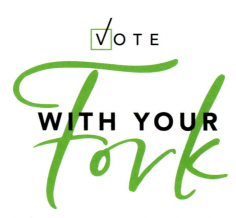

☑ VOTE WITH YOUR *Fork*

It's never been easier to make plant-based choices. Just about every restaurant in the world now caters to vegans and every day, new places are popping up in every city that have fully plant-based menus. The grocery store has entire aisles now dedicated to meat and dairy substitutes and there are hundreds of blogs and instagram accounts with unbelievable vegan recipes. Of course the vegan cookbook world has completely taken off as well. So I am 100% confident that with a little trial and error, you can enjoy a fully plant-based lifestyle without ever compromising your taste buds.

As I stated previously, I believe in progress over perfection. If you can incorporate even one plant-based meal a day, I applaud you. A meatless day a week? Again, I applaud you. Every little choice you make is a vote for the planet—currently our only home. A vote for your health, you only have one body, afterall. And a vote for the animals, who have no voice of their own. I am so happy to celebrate any and all plant-based choices. In a perfect world, I would love to see a plant-based world with only choices that support the health of humanity and the Earth, but I'm so thankful for you and every single plant-based option you adopt into your nutritional philosophy in whatever way feels best for you.

I certainly wasn't raised this way by any stretch of the imagination, but I'm thankful that I found it. It's been an incredible journey for me. Having to completely relearn everything I thought I knew about food, nutrition, my repertoire of recipes and my entire lifestyle. It didn't happen overnight, rather it was an aggregate of small choices over the years that lead me to fully embracing this lifestyle 100%. Every step of the way I was rewarded. The more I shifted towards a plant-based diet, the better I felt in my body, my mind and my spirit.

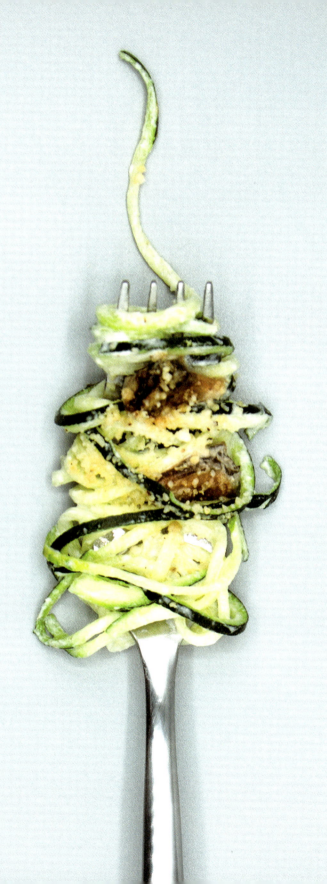

WHY PLANT-BASED? 23

WHY Juice?

Juicing changed my life, so it's no wonder I decided to share juicing with the world through my cafés (Choice Superfood Bar and Juicery), along with all the other delicious meals we serve. In fact, I remember the first time I did a cleanse and let me just say, I definitely had moments of serious doubt in my decision making abilities (what was I thinking?). Initially it was really hard and I felt deprived of all the things I loved: bread, cheese, bread, pasta… did I mention bread?

But seriously, choosing to commit to that 21-day cleanse was one of the best decisions in my life. I juiced and ate mostly raw fruits and vegetables for the entire 3 weeks! I never knew the power of juice until then.

While I had always enjoyed a green juice here and there because it made me feel good, I never really knew what it was doing inside my cells, and how that affected me overall. I never knew how bad I felt until going through the process of cleaning out my system and feeling the shift on a deep, cellular level.

Committing to 21-days fully plant-based taught me what it felt like to feel good in my mind and body - and have the energy of a toddler on a sugar high (without all the caffeine and other junk!). I found myself craving green things after that cleanse was over, like salads and vegetables, and more fresh juice.

When I reached day 22, and had my first "heavy" meal in weeks, I felt awful. And as strange as it may sound, that was actually a huge gift! In the past, I didn't pay much attention as to how I felt when I ate poorly because it had become my "normal" state. But after feeling so good for multiple weeks in a row, anything less than that was obvious!

Feeling good became a priority, which meant it became much easier to start shifting my diet to one that consisted of lots of organic plant-based foods and cold-pressed juices. One of the things I learned from that experience was that juice (specifically, organic, cold-pressed juice) has up to 6 pounds of organic produce per serving! When was the last time you sat down and ate 6 pounds of produce? Yeah, I can't remember either! Imagine all of those enzymes, minerals and vitamins flooding your system - and tasting amazing as well! That's some seriously potent juice if you ask me. Cleansing on occasion, and juicing daily changed my body on a cellular level. And over time, it literally changed my life.

We have all heard the saying, "You are what you eat." But what most people don't realize is that we also begin to crave what we eat. So making juicing (and other healthy choices) part of your daily routine is far more powerful than you may have given it credit for.

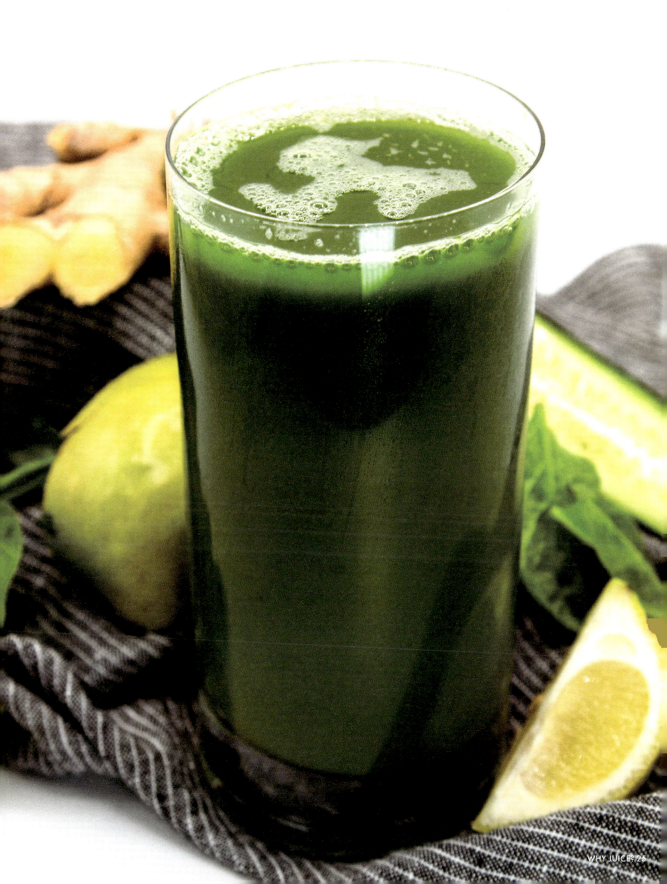

6 REASONS YOU SHOULD DRINK JUICE EVERY DAY

#1. IT'S ALKALIZING FOR THE BODY

All organic matter (including soil, plants and animals) can be represented by their pH level. **pH** stands for Potential of Hydrogen and is the ratio measurement between acid and alkaline. Maintaining a balanced pH level in the body is critical for achieving and maintaining long-term *optimal* health. Unfortunately for many of us, many of the foods we eat are acidic - particularly diets high in animal protein because meat favors the acidic side of the pH scale. Even common things like coffee and alcohol are acidic so enjoying in moderation is definitely recommended. Fresh pressed juice (not the store bought stuff that's been sitting on the shelves for who knows how long) is a powerful alkalizing agent, which can help the body achieve a balanced pH.

#2. PROVIDES SUSTAINED ENERGY

By upping your vitamin and mineral intake, **your body naturally assimilates and utilizes REAL nutrients,** to keep your energy balanced throughout the day. Caffeinated beverages can be tough on your hard-working body, and often lead to spikes and dips (the good ol' afternoon crash).

#3. ANTI-AGING

Juicing floods your system with antioxidants, which protect you from oxidative damage, the primary contributor to physical aging (like those pesky fine lines and wrinkles).

#4. IMPROVED GUT HEALTH

We now know that your gut is the foundation of health. In fact, studies even show that it can mean the difference between depression and happiness. It affects nearly every aspect of your health, which is why it's crucial to take the steps necessary to ensure your gut is in optimal health. Drinking green juice supports your body from the inside out.

#5. ENHANCED DETOXIFICATION

By consuming green juice every day, you're giving your liver a fighting chance against all the toxins you're exposed to on a daily basis. Even if you eat a clean diet, our environment is full of junk, which we're absorbing through our skin and the air we breathe.

#6. IMMUNE BOOSTING

Green juice is one of the best ways to support a healthy immune system because it's packed full of nutrition. Drinking a green juice every day is an easy way to replenish the nutrients your immune system needs to keep you feeling (and looking) your best.

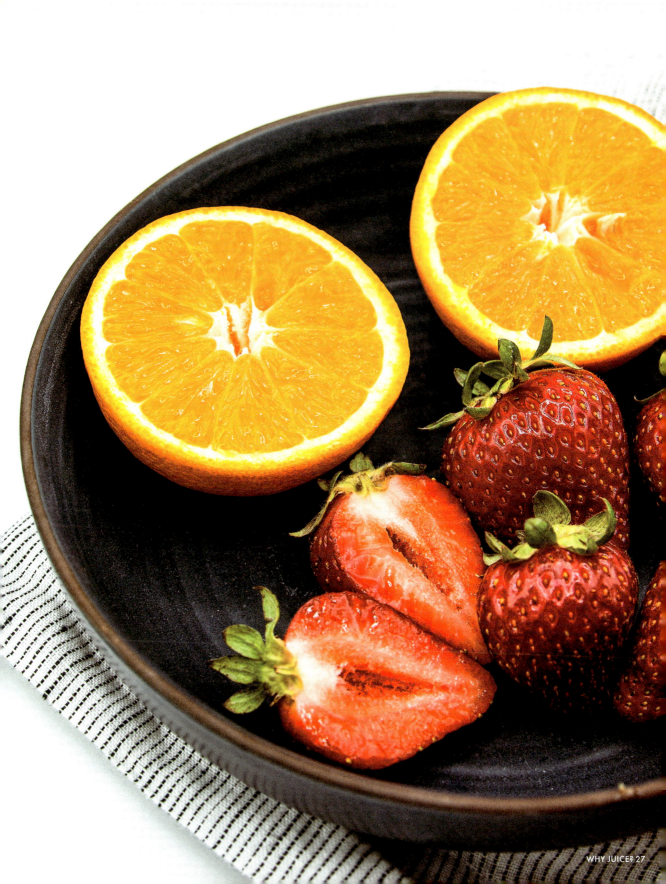

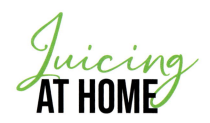
Juicing AT HOME

So now that we've established some of the amazing benefits of incorporating fresh pressed juice into our daily regimen, let's talk about how to make it happen. Of course, popping into Choice to pick up a cold-pressed juice is a great option—chock-full of organic goodness without any of the work that juicing on your own involves. But we know that's not realistic or sustainable for most people on a daily basis. That being said, juicing at home is a great option when you have the time in your schedule (and I promise, it's actually not that complicated!). But there are a few things you should definitely consider...

Type of Juicer: CENTRIFUGE vs. COLD-PRESS

CENTRIFUGAL machines tend to be more affordable, entry-level juicers. These juicers extract juice using a spinning metal blade, which produces heat and friction. While it's true that the heat oxidizes the nutrients and destroys some of the enzymes in your produce, you're still left with some really incredible nutrients to fuel your body with. This option is better than nothing at all!

If you opt to use a centrifuge, you'll want to consume the juice immediately after juicing your produce to get the most benefit. Because of how this machine works, the nutrients in the juice will continue to decline as time goes on making immediate consumption your best bet. It's important to note: there's not as much bang for your buck when it comes to juicing those leafy greens in these juicers either. You'll lose a lot of potential juice in the process with these appliances.

COLD-PRESSED JUICE protects and preserves the nutrients of the fruits and vegetables. Since the cold press juicer presses the produce to extract the juice, no heat or friction is involved, which means you get 100% of the vitamins, minerals, enzymes, and nutrients when you drink cold-pressed juice vs. store bought brands that over time, turn to sugar.

And bonus: You can store cold-pressed juice for up to 5 days (depending on the juice). The nutrition in cold-pressed juice stays intact, unlike it's centrifuge juice counterparts.

As if higher quality nutrition wasn't enough of a reason to make cold-pressed juice a part of your daily life, it also just so happens to taste better.

There are a lot of affordable in-home slow, cold-press juicers that will give you a higher quality juice and a longer shelf life, allowing you to bulk up on those juice days and stock your fridge for the week.

Rub-A-Dub-Dub, Give That Produce A Scrub

Even though I recommend juicing only organic fruits and vegetables, it's possible that some sneaky critters (like bugs, bacteria, and other parasites) might be lingering. Give your produce a good scrub before you put it through the juicer, so you can feel good about sipping on that organic goodness.

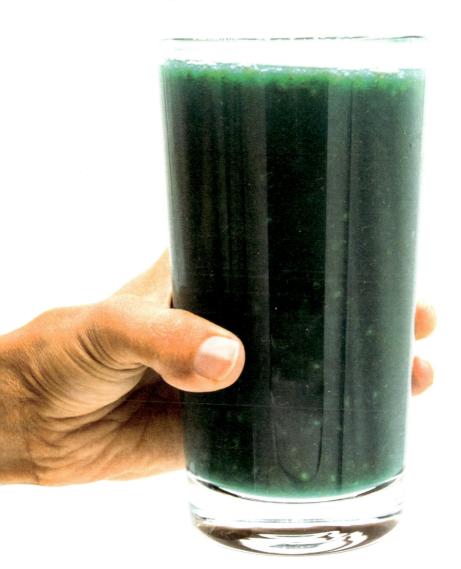

__NOTE__:
Produce is constantly changing based on seasonality, where it's grown, and even how it's grown. Because of the potential variables due to the above, be mindful when you are juicing and following juice recipes. It's a good practice to always add individual ingredients a little at a time, so you can adjust to taste as you go.

ONLY USE ORGANIC PRODUCE
(ANYTHING ELSE IS A PESTICIDE COCKTAIL!)

If you are NOT going to juice 100% organic, you may be causing yourself more harm than good. Juice is 100% absorbed in your body within minutes of being consumed. If the produce being juiced is not organic, all the other chemicals in or on the plant (pesticides, fungicides, herbicides, synthetic fertilizers) will also be part of the juice. Even if you wash conventional produce, you must understand that the pesticides used in the process are absorbed into the plant itself, so washing will not fully prevent you from consuming the pesticides.

All that aside, supporting the organic movement is so important to our environmental sustainability. Every purchase you make is a vote. Please vote organic every time—for your health and for the planet. Yes, it may cost a little more, but I want to encourage you to think about your health as the investment that it is. Organic produce is cheaper than a trip to the ER! And you are so worth investing in!

Keep It Cold

One of our favorite sayings in the Choice kitchen is "keep it cold and keep it clean." It's so important to keep juice cold when working with raw produce. You may be up to your eyeballs in kale and apple pulp and be tempted to leave fresh juice out while you continue to juice other produce. . .it's easy to want to blow through the rest of the juicing and get the job done so you can move on with your day. Don't do it! For the best result and the longest shelf life of each ingredient—keep it cold! Juice each ingredient separately, refrigerating as you move onto the next ingredient, before combining everything together and enjoying your delicious and nutritious recipe!

Don't Lean, CLEAN

Another saying we have at Choice is, "if you've got time to lean, you've got time to clean." Let's be honest, the cleanup is really the only part about juicing at home that pretty much sucks. Juicers are made up of multiple parts, and the pulp has a tendency to get everywhere! Take it from me though, you want to wash your juicer as soon as you're done with it! The longer you let that pulp sit there, the harder it will be to get it cleaned up! So no leaning (and lagging) after you make your yummy goodness - get to cleaning the moment you've finished.

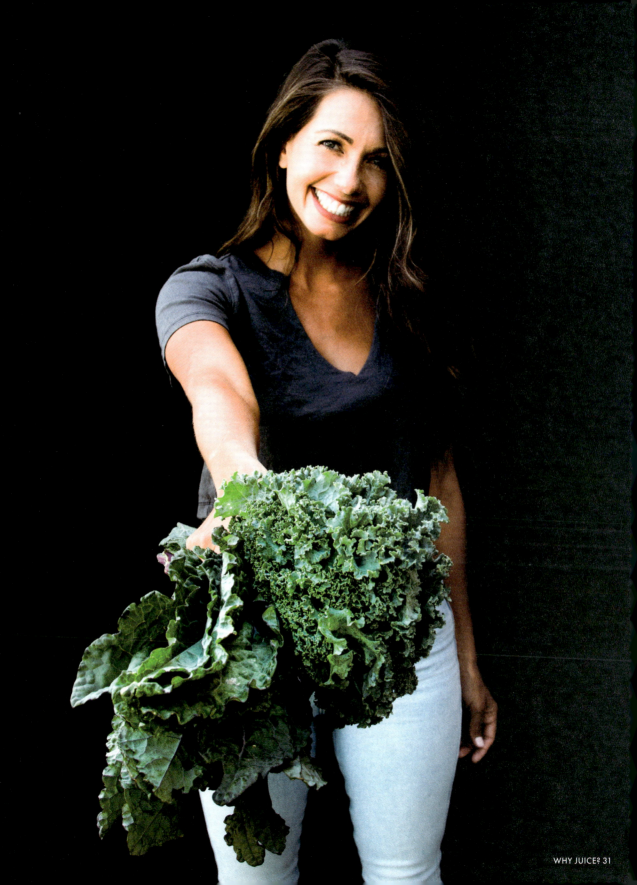

Super Foods FOR SUPER HUMANS

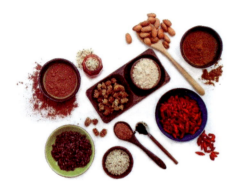

According to Google, a superfood is "a nutrient-rich food considered to be especially beneficial for health and well-being." Great, but what does that really mean?

To put it simply, superfoods are nutritional powerhouses! Superfoods are extremely high in micronutrients like vitamins, minerals, as well as antioxidants, enzymes and healthy fats. All of these nutrients are essential to your body so you can thrive.

Superfoods are the superheroes of the plant world. While some superheroes are out fighting crime, these superheroes are fueling our bodies on a cellular level so our bodies can more easily ward off chronic disease, aging, and other nutrient deficiencies.

You will find a lot of superfoods included in the recipes in this book. There are so many superfoods, I could probably fill an entire book talking about them. But for the intents and purposes of this recipe book, I've included only a few of my favorites. If you aren't already familiar with some (or all) of them, I encourage you to spend some time researching the incredible superpowers of the world's most nutrient dense foods. Below, I've included many of the superfoods that are also included in the recipes to follow. You can also find all of these superfoods on our yummy menu at Choice.

The word 'superfood' has become quite the buzzword and is often thrown around lightly thanks to clever marketing campaigns - but what makes a food so super?

ALMONDS
Almonds contain lots of healthy fats, fiber, protein, magnesium and vitamin E. Health benefits may include lower blood sugar levels, reduced blood pressure, and lower cholesterol levels. They may also reduce hunger and promote weight loss.

ASHWAGANDHA
Ashwagandha is an ancient medicinal herb that has been shown to reduce blood sugar levels, and symptoms of depression. It also has been shown to be effective in reducing stress and anxiety.

ACAÍ
Acaí berries are grape-like fruits native to the rainforests of South America, and are harvested from acaí palm trees. They are one of the most antioxidant-rich fruits in the world. Due to the high levels of antioxidants, they have powerful heart healing properties. Acaí can reduce the risks of Alzheimer's disease and macular degeneration. This means prevention of cardiovascular disease, improvement in eyesight and lots of other anti-aging benefits. Not to mention, acaí can increase blood circulation and lower the risk of blood clots.

BAOBAB
The baobab fruit and powder are rich in vitamin C, potassium, carbohydrates, phosphorus, pectins, calcium, and iron. It has antimicrobial, antiviral, antioxidant, and anti-inflammatory properties. Baobab is native to Madagascar, Australia, and Africa and is one of nature's oldest trees.

BLUE MAJIK
Blue Majik is rich in iron, vitamin B12 and vitamin A. Clinical research suggests that Blue Majik may promote; support of healthy inflammation responses after exercise, support of healthy joints and flexibility, support for antioxidant and cellular protection, increased energy, vitality and endurance.

CACAO (POWDER AND NIBS)
Cacao is said to mean "food of the gods," as it is loaded with antioxidants and is one of the highest sources of magnesium, which is essential for muscle and nerve function. Cacao is also a good source of fiber, protein, healthy fats and iron. Cacao can raise energy levels, improve cognitive function, and elevate your mood among many other benefits.

CAMU CAMU
The camu camu berry is a red, cherry-like fruit that grows in small bushy riverside trees from the Amazon rainforest in Peru and Brazil. Camu camu is antimicrobial, anti-inflammatory and is an antioxidant. It has been shown to increase energy and is used to maintain healthy gums, eyes, and skin, and to stimulate the immune system.

CHAGA MUSHROOM
Chaga mushrooms contain a wide variety of vitamins, minerals, and nutrients. Benefits may include slowing the aging process, lowering cholesterol, preventing and fighting cancer, lowering blood pressure, supporting the immune system, fighting inflammation and lowering blood sugar.

CHIA SEEDS
Chia seeds are one of the most nutritious foods on the planet. They are loaded with fiber, protein, and omega-3 fatty acids. Chia seeds high fiber and protein content are great for increased satiety (they keep you feeling fuller, longer). They are also high in calcium, magnesium, and phosphorus which are essential for bone health.

GOJI BERRIES
Goji berries are bright orange-red in color, and are one of the most nutritionally dense fruits on Earth. They provides immune system support and may protect against cancer. Goji berries promote healthy skin, stabilize blood sugar, improve depression, anxiety, and sleep and can prevent liver damage.

HEMP SEEDS
Hemp seeds are a great source of protein and omega-3 fatty acids, which are good for heart health. They also contain fiber, potassium, iron, zinc, and B vitamins, and may reduce inflammation, lower cholesterol and blood pressure. Hemp seeds aid in rapid recovery from disease or injury, and help with natural blood sugar control. Hemp seeds have also been shown to help with weight loss and increased and sustained energy.

LION'S MANE MUSHROOM
Lion's mane mushrooms are white, globe-shaped fungi that have long, shaggy spines. Health benefits may include reduced inflammation and improved cognitive and heart health. Lion's mane mushrooms may enhance the immune system, partly by reducing inflammation and preventing oxidation. Lion's mane encourages the growth of beneficial gut bacteria that strengthen immunity, and has been shown to be beneficial in the treatment of anxiety and depression.

LUCUMA
Lucuma is a subtropical fruit native to Peru. It has a sweet, cake-like flavor and while it is a sweetener, it does not have an effect on the glycemic index (meaning, no dips and spikes - or crashes). Lucuma is also high in vitamin B3 and other B vitamins.

MACA
Maca is a root and is nutritionally rich with vitamins and minerals (vitamins B, C, and E and calcium, zinc, and iron). Maca may boost libido and increase endurance. It is known for its hormone balancing affects, and may increase fertility, and relieve menstrual issues.

MULBERRIES
Mulberries are colorful berries that are eaten both fresh and dried. They're a good source of iron, vitamin C, and fiber, making mulberries great for digestive health. They may boost metabolism, aid in red blood cell production, support the immune system, and are anti-aging.

REISHI MUSHROOM
Reishi mushroom has been used to help enhance the immune system, reduce stress, improve sleep, and lessen fatigue. People also take reishi mushroom for health conditions such as: high blood pressure, high cholesterol, cardiovascular disease, liver or kidney disease, respiratory diseases (such as asthma), viral infections (such as the flu), HIV/AIDS, cancer and support during chemotherapy, and for building strength and stamina.

TURMERIC
The most powerful anti-inflammatory on the planet! Health benefits may include the potential to prevent heart disease, Alzheimer's, cancer, arthritis, and can improve symptoms of depression. Turmeric is also associated with improved brain function and may lower the risk of brain disease.

CHAPTER 3

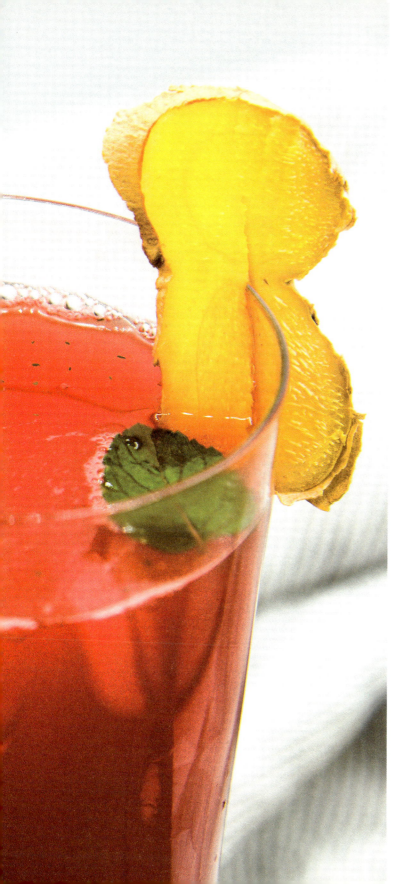

JUICES

There is so much juice available in today's world. Just take a stroll down your local health food store aisles and you will see the shelves lined with a myriad of varieties! And for many of us (at least in California), there seems to be a juice shop on every corner (which is great!). But sadly, a lot of juice (most, actually) has been through a pasteurization process in order to get onto those shelves. That process extends the shelf life upwards of 45 days, but lowers the nutritional value and integrity of the juice. Total bummer.

If you have access to a local organic juicery that offers raw, certified organic juice, that's fabulous! There are so many benefits to buying raw, organic, cold-pressed juice (aside from the delicious taste). The biggest bonus to buying your juice is that you're cutting out all the work of juicing at home, not to mention the clean up. That being said, it does get pricey so it's nice to learn how to make some delicious juice recipes at home. Always remember, it's important to buy quality which means, choosing organic produce and using a slow juicer if possible (see Chapter 2 for more info on the topic).

SWEET GREENS

This is one of my favorite green juices. It's simple, it's green and it's just the perfect amount of sweet. This is very similar to our most popular green juice, Choice Greens.

INGREDIENTS:

1 ¼ CUP
Kale Juice

¼ CUP
Spinach Juice

½ CUP
Apple Juice

1 CUP
Cucumber Juice

1 TBSP
Lemon Juice

1 TSP
Ginger Juice

BENEFITS:

This juice is chock-full of healing and cleansing compounds. That being said, the belle of the ball in this juice is definitely kale. Of all the healthy greens, kale is king. It is definitely one of the healthiest and most nutritious plant foods in existence. Kale is loaded with all sorts of beneficial compounds, some of which have powerful medicinal properties. Kale is loaded with vitamin A, K, C, B6, manganese, calcium, copper, potassium and magnesium. Kale is high in powerful antioxidants like quercetin and kaempferol, and contains substances that have been shown to help fight cancer.

TRIFECTA

This is an OG Choice green juice. With just three ingredients, it's so easy to make! Let's be honest, when juicing at home—simplicity is everything. What's also great about this juice is that it's pure greens with no sweet added (yet still delicious). A lot of juicers out there prefer to take their greens straight up! Kudos to them. I don't mind having sugar from fruit in my juices, though I do appreciate a pure green juice from time to time. I love making this one at home on the days I can't get into one of the shops.

INGREDIENTS:

1 CUP
Celery Juice

1 CUP
Cucumber Juice

¼ CUP
Kale Juice

SPLASH OF
Lemon Juice

BENEFITS:

We have already covered the healing powers of kale in the recipe above, so here we are going to focus on celery juice. There's been a lot of buzz around celery juice, and for good reason. Celery seems to be the newest holy grail of healing drinks - and I'm a huge fan of the celery detox. Let's be clear, celery is awesome! That's because it's a plant, and every plant has its own unique benefits. Celery contains impressive amounts of vitamins C and K as well as folate and potassium. Recent studies have found celery juice to be particularly great for helping to fight cancer and liver disease, reduce inflammation (especially for brain related diseases) and boost cardiovascular health.

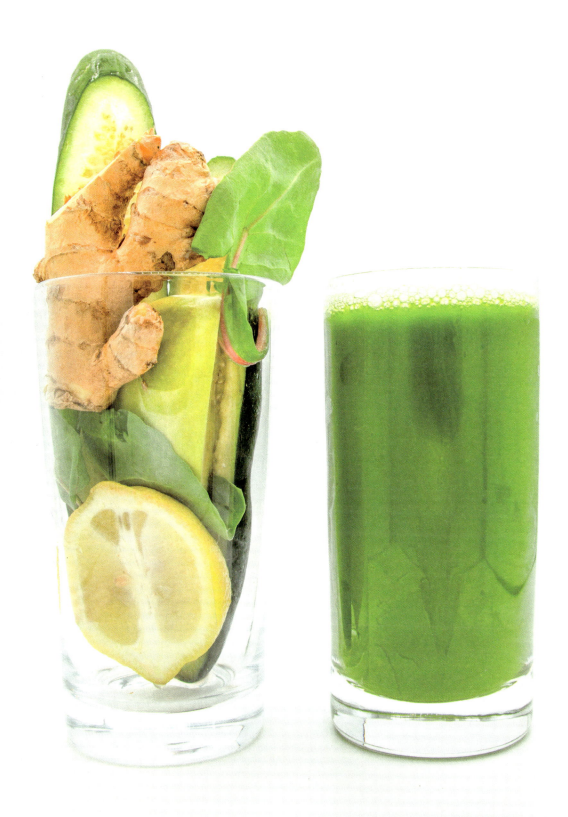

STARBURST (JUICE)

This is another easy-to-make juice that will leave you feeling that burst of energy for hours to come.

INGREDIENTS:

½ CUP
Strawberry Juice

½ CUP
Orange Juice

1 CUP
Pineapple Juice

1 ½ TSP
Lime Juice

1 TBSP
Mint, blended and strained (OPTIONAL)

OPTIONAL ADD-IN:

For a fresh hint of mint, add 1 Tbsp of fresh mint leaves to ½ cup of juice and blend in a high powered blender for about 5 seconds, then strain and add back to the remaining juice. Yum!

BENEFITS:

This juice is loaded with vitamin C and a plethora of other antioxidants, vitamins and minerals. Strawberries are particularly high in folate and potassium. This is a great juice to drink regularly to keep your immunity up. If you feel like you're coming down with something, try drinking a fresh, vitamin C potent beverage (instead of store bought powders promising to heal your body). You'll be so glad you did!

STRAWBERRY SUNRISE

If you are a Choice regular, maybe you've had our Hot Sunrise. What you may not know is that Hot Sunrise was originally made with strawberry juice, not pineapple. Strawberry is very seasonal so we used to change it up seasonally, and the pineapple version eventually took over. This is the non-spicy version of our original Hot Sunrise. If you want to spice it up, add a touch of cayenne.

INGREDIENTS:

2 TSP
Lime Juice

½ CUP
Strawberry Juice

1 TSP
Ginger Juice

1 CUP
Coconut Water

¾ CUP
Orange Juice

(OPTIONAL)
ADD ¼ – ½ TSP
Cayenne
to make this a Spicy Strawberry Sunrise

BENEFITS:

The coconut water in this recipe is very hydrating and great for replenishing electrolytes, making this an awesome post-workout beverage. Strawberries are very high in anti-oxidants, as well as folate and potassium. Ginger is among the healthiest (and in my opinion, most delicious) spices on the planet. It is loaded with nutrients and bioactive compounds that have powerful benefits for your body and brain. Ginger has a very long history of use in various forms of traditional and alternative medicine. It has been used to help digestion, reduce nausea, fight the flu, and the common cold, just to name a few things. The orange in this recipe lends to more than just the incredible taste. It's high vitamin C content helps with immune boosting benefits as well as promoting healthy skin and contributes to its potential anti-cancer properties.

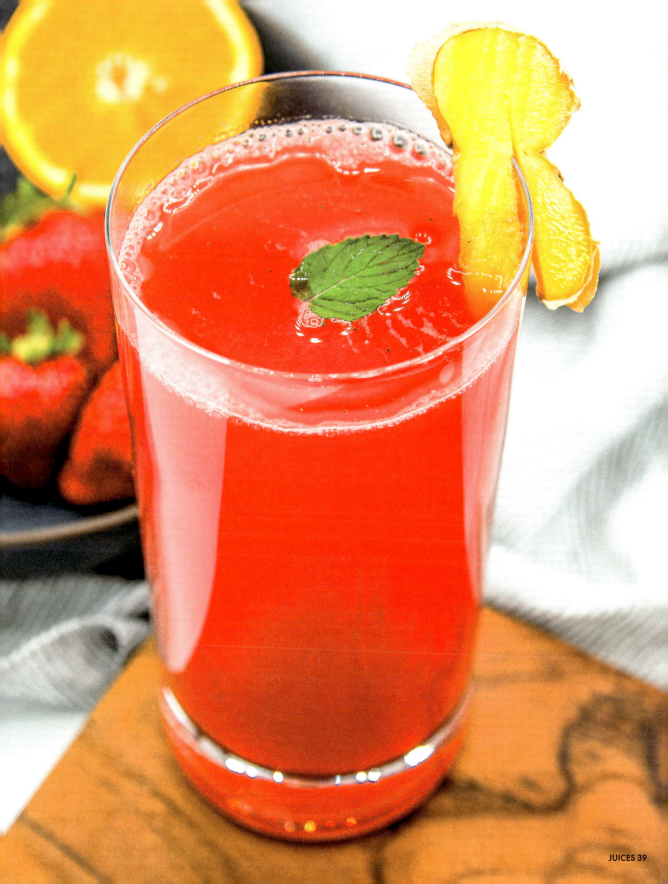

BEET CHIA TROPIC

This is similar to our famous Beet Chia, but with a tropical spin. We've incorporated pineapple, which is great for digestion, among many other things (see the benefits list below). Pineapple can be on the sweet side, so you can get more beets into this recipe without compromising the flavor.

INGREDIENTS:

¾-1 CUP
Beet Juice

¾ CUP
Pineapple Juice

1 TSP
Ginger Juice

2 OZ
Chia Gel
(1 ½ tsp chia seeds soaked in ¼ cup water for 30 mins)

¼ CUP
Orange Juice

1 ½ TSP
Lemon Juice

BENEFITS:

Beet juice is known for its ability to increase stamina, reduce inflammation, lower blood pressure and combat anemia. Ginger is known to boost brain function and lower blood sugar. Pineapple has a plethora of benefits but in this juice, we are focusing on the immune system support, bone strength and anti-inflammatory properties.

Beets can be pretty hard to get down with their strong earthy taste, but pairing them with pineapple and ginger helps to balance this juice making it a tasty (and powerful) combo.

The chia is added into the mix for it's high fiber content, which helps your body to regulate insulin levels. Chia also happens to be a great source of protein, fiber and omega-3s.

NOTE:

Chia is better when soaked! If you soak them, then you sprout them, which releases the enzyme inhibitors that are used to protect the seed. This makes it much easier to digest and your body can then access the dense nutrients inside the seeds. In my opinion, you always want to get the most nutrition out of any food that you eat, so I prefer soaking them before adding them to my recipes or smoothies, if possible. Either way, they're still an excellent source of nutrition.

How to soak your chia seeds: Add 1 ½ tsp chia seeds to ¼ cup water for a minimum of 30 mins up to overnight. This makes 2 oz of chia gel.

> "You always want to get the most nutrition out of any food that you eat."

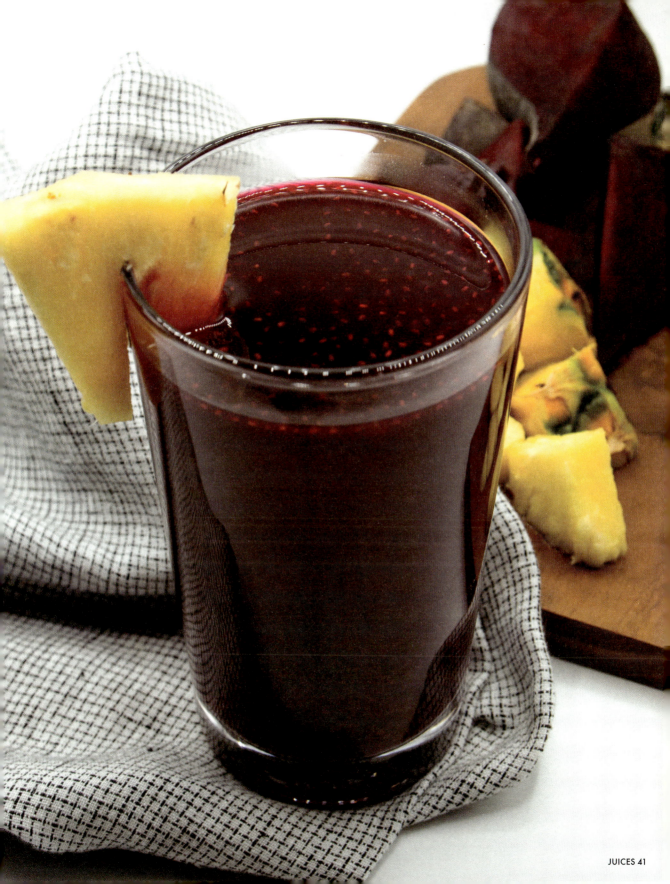

AVATAR

This is one of my all time favorite juices. The cucumber in this recipe makes it so refreshing and hydrating. The pineapple lends to it's sweet, tropical flavor, and the chia makes it very filling. And the Blue Majik (ohhhhh the MAGIC) really packs a serious nutritional punch. This is a great post workout beverage both for hydration and muscle recovery.

INGREDIENTS:

1 CUP
Pineapple Juice

1 CUP
Cucumber Juice

1 TSP
E3Live Blue Majik

2 TBSP
Chia Gel (1 oz)

BENEFITS:

This juice is a great source of omega-3s, protein, fiber, and antioxidants. Plus, it's alkalizing, great for muscle repair, boosts digestion and hydration. Speaking of Blue Majik specifically, research shows phycocyanin, the active pigment-protein complex in blue spirulina, can remove heavy metals, protect cells from DNA damage caused by aging and the environment and reduce disease-causing inflammation throughout the body. It also helps boost immunity, encourages an ideal pH balance and is rich in beautifying minerals.

SKINNY COOLER

Not only is this juice hydrating, alkalizing and detoxifying, it's also absolutely delicious. I love a little kick in my juice and the jalapeño in this recipe delivers just that. This is a great post workout juice because it's incredibly hydrating and has plenty of electrolytes to replenish you after any strenuous activity. You can adjust the jalapeño to get your desired kick (or eliminate it altogether if you're not really a spicy-juice lover)!

Pineapple is high in antioxidants and great for digestion. Cucumber is extremely hydrating, and is known to aid in weight loss while also containing antioxidants, and anti-inflammatory properties. The jalapeños in this juice are also great for weight loss due to the chemical capsaicin, which is what actually gives them their hot properties. Capsaicin also acts as an anti-inflammatory, which makes it great for reducing swelling and pain in those who suffer from arthritis. Another cool benefit of this miracle chemical is that it can actually help to ease pain, specifically related to headaches. Capsaicin in peppers actually blocks the neuropeptide known as substance P, which is the main pain transmitter to the brain. Jalapeños are also great for lowering blood pressure!

INGREDIENTS:

1 CUP
Cucumber Juice

1 CUP
Pineapple Juice

¼ - ½ TSP
Jalapeño (SEE NOTE)

1 TBSP
Mint, blended and strained

OPTIONAL ADD-IN :

For that spicy kick, add ¼ - ½ tsp chopped jalapeño (and 1 Tbsp of fresh mint leaves - optional) to ½ cup of juice and blend in a high powered blender for about 5 seconds, then strain and add back to the remaining juice. Yum!

NOTE:

I like it spicy and typically that's accomplished with ½ tsp, but I always start with ¼ and add to taste. Jalapeños vary in spice, so it's important to add a little at a time and taste as you go.

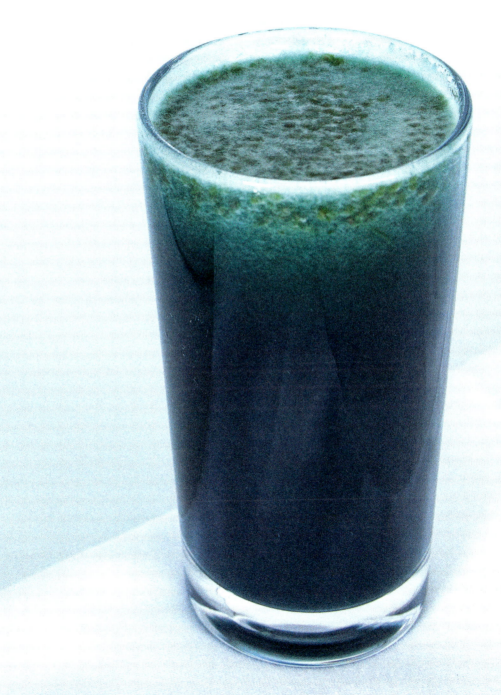

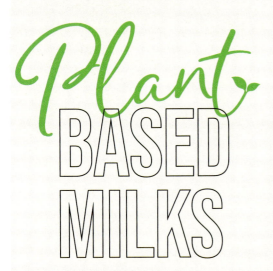

Plant-BASED MILKS

For the sake of this book, I'm going to focus on my personal favorites, offering easy to make at home recipes that can be whipped up in under 10 minutes (minus soaking time).

THE DIRTY OF DAIRY

Dairy is scary - and the global decline of dairy sales just goes to show that the word is out. It's highly acidic to the body, so much so that it can actually leach calcium from the bones. It's high in saturated fat and it's been linked to heart disease and a variety of cancers. Not to mention the fact that nearly 75% of the world's population is genetically unable to properly digest cow's milk and other dairy products. Yikes. So much for "milk does a body good," right? The dairy industry is also highly unsustainable and it's definitely not cruelty free. With all of the incredible alternatives available, it's never been easier to make the switch.

SO LET'S CHAT OPTIONS...

ALMOND MILK

This is a very healthy milk-substitute. It contains lots of vitamins, magnesium, iron, protein and fiber. Plus, it's naturally very creamy! It's important to soak/sprout your almonds before making your milk. This breaks down all the enzyme inhibitors making the nutrients in the almonds more bioavailable (easier for your body to assimilate).

COCONUT MILK

Often praised for it's health benefits, coconut milk is a crowd pleaser. Naturally creamy with a sweet nutty flavor, it's known to strengthen the immune system due to the lauric acid, a medium chain fatty acid in the coconut flesh, which exhibits antimicrobial and anti-cancer properties. It's also known for its MCTs (medium chain triglycerides) that have been shown to fuel your brain and boost cognitive function. The coconut water used in making the coconut milk provides large doses of potassium, magnesium, calcium, sodium and other electrolytes that are great for hydration and athletic performance, as well as your overall health.

HEMP MILK

Hemp seeds are one of the highest sources of plant-based protein. Hemp seeds are also naturally high in omega-3s, alpha-linolenic acid (ALA) and have the ideal ratio of omega 3 to omega 6 essential fatty acids (1:3) to promote brain and heart health. Plus, hemp seeds are a good source of magnesium, iron, vitamin B1 and calcium. Hemp milk actually contains more calcium than it's dairy counterpart!

OAT MILK

Oat milk is a sensible option for those with dietary restrictions. Since it's made from just oats and water, it's vegan and free of nuts and soy. Oat milk is low in fat and contains no cholesterol. It's nutritional benefits include vitamin A, fiber, calcium and iron.

NOTE:

All of these varieties are available commercially at just about any supermarket all over the world. So you may be asking, why would I make these myself? Making your own "milk" at home gives you the power to decide what ingredients are going in your "milk" and how much, so you have full control over the sugar content without any additives, preservatives or thickening agents. Of course, homemade means it will also be raw and will not have gone through any type of pasteurization process that may otherwise compromise the integrity of its nutrition profile.

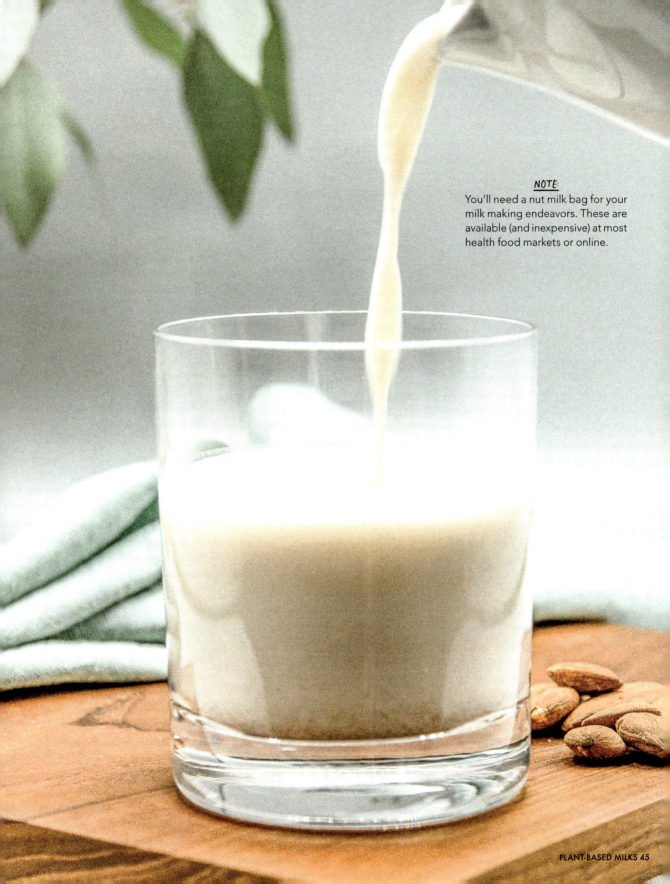

NOTE:
You'll need a nut milk bag for your milk making endeavors. These are available (and inexpensive) at most health food markets or online.

SOAK THOSE NUTS AND SEEDS

Nuts and seeds, like grains, contain protective agents (inhibitors) that protect them and prevent them from germinating until the conditions are perfect. When these foods are ingested, their protective agents act as enzyme inhibitors in our bodies which can compromise our digestion and interfere with nutrient absorption.

Soaking nuts and seeds essentially replicates the perfect moist conditions required for germination and neutralizes these anti-nutrients and enzyme inhibitors, making them more easily digestible and making the nutrition in the nuts and seeds more bioavailable.

Soaking your nuts and seeds helps to unlock nutrients, makes digestion easier, and improves the flavor and texture of the nuts and seeds (the texture is especially important when making things like nut milks, cheeses, sauces, etc.).

Take your soaking a step further with

Sprouting

Soaking and sprouting your nuts and seeds takes them from a dormant seed and turns them into *live plants*. Pretty cool, right? Only truly raw nuts and seeds will sprout. At Choice, we have to import our almonds from another country because almonds from the U.S. are all pasteurized (which is one of the many reasons our smoothies are so incredible!). We use only raw organic almonds, which we then soak to begin the sprouting process, activating these little nutrient powerhouses and turning the active almonds into our almond milk, the base of every smoothie and bowl in our shops. There is a lot of information available online about sprouting the different nuts and seeds so if this sounds interesting to you, I encourage you to dive in further.

HERE'S WHAT YOU'LL NEED TO
Sprout your Almonds

- 2 cups of raw almonds
- Filtered water
- Quart mason jar with lid
- Cheesecloth
- Small bowl

METHOD FOR SPROUTING:

01. Place almonds into a quart mason jar. Fill with filtered water and cover with a cheesecloth, securing with just the ring of the lid so they can still breathe. Allow the jar to sit on the counter overnight. The next morning, remove the cheesecloth and drain the water from the quart jar. Fill the jar again with fresh filtered water, swirl the almonds, and drain the water. Replace the cheesecloth and, using a small bowl, store the jar upside down at an angle so excess water can drain out and air can circulate inside the jar.

02. Repeat the above step each morning and night until the almonds begin to sprout.

03. Once all the nuts are sprouted, store them in a jar in the fridge for a few days or dehydrate them to store longer. The sprout itself will look different depending on what seed or nut you're sprouting.

Recipe time!

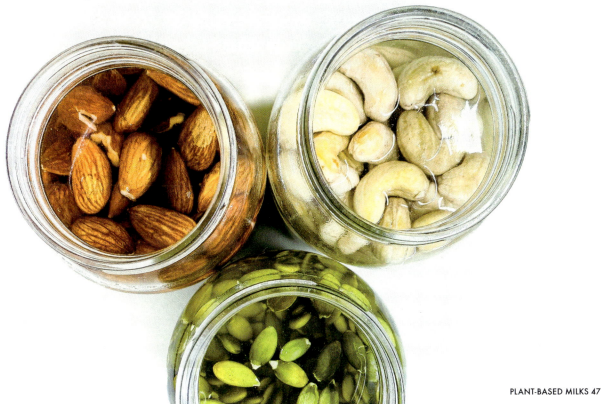

SPROUTED VANILLA ALMOND MILK

INGREDIENTS:

1 CUP
Sprouted Almonds
(see directions above)

4 CUPS
Water

2 LARGE
Medjool Dates, pitted

1 TSP
Pure Vanilla Extract

1 PINCH
Himalayan Salt

PREPARATION:

01. Combine all of the ingredients in a high speed blender and blend for approximately 2 minutes. Carefully strain the mixture through a nut milk bag and set pulp aside for use in other recipes (or discard).

02. Transfer to a sealed container and refrigerate. Will keep in the refrigerator up to 5 days (sometimes more).

03. Shake well before using.

STRAWBERRY MILK

INGREDIENTS:

Use the *Sprouted Vanilla Almond Milk* recipe above
(4 CUPS), then add:

6 LARGE
Medjool Dates, pitted

2 CUPS
Frozen Strawberries

1 PINCH
Himalayan Salt

PREPARATION:

01. Add 6 dates, 2 cups of frozen or fresh strawberries and a pinch of Himalayan salt to 4 cups of Sprouted Vanilla Almond Milk.

02. Blend on high speed for about 2 minutes, or until strawberries and dates are blended thoroughly. Refrigerate immediately until you are ready to enjoy. You can add more dates or strawberries depending on how sweet you want your milk.

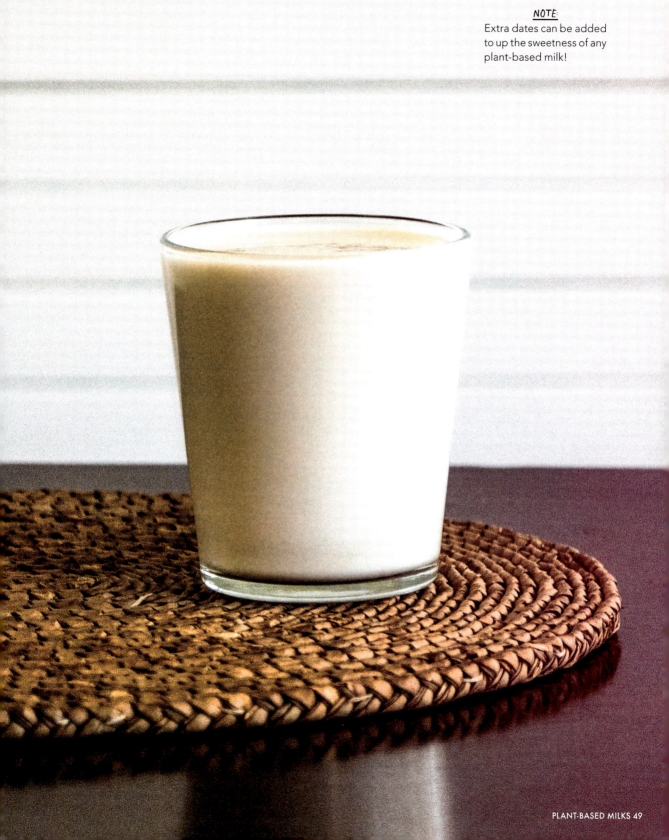

NOTE: Extra dates can be added to up the sweetness of any plant-based milk!

COCONUT MILK

INGREDIENTS:

4 CUPS
Coconut Water
(from fresh young coconut)

¾ CUP
Young Coconut Meat
(scooped from coconut)

1 TBSP
Coconut Butter, packed

⅜ TSP
Himalayan Salt

PREPARATION:

01. Combine all of the ingredients in a high speed blender and blend for approximately 1-2 minutes. Carefully strain the mixture through a nut milk bag and discard the pulp. You won't have much pulp with this recipe, but feel free to store it and use it in any way your heart desires. I toss mine into smoothies, oatmeal or into baked goods.

02. Transfer to a sealed container and refrigerate. Will keep in the refrigerator up to 5 days (sometimes more). Shake well before using.

MAJIK MILK

INGREDIENTS:

Use the *Coconut Milk* recipe above
(4 CUPS), then add:

2 TSP
E3Live Blue Majik

PREPARATION:

01. Follow instructions for coconut milk recipe above. Add in Blue Majik and blend for 20 seconds.

NOTE:
Not familiar with Blue Majik? You should be! Blue Majik is jam-packed with nutrients such as protein, B vitamins (including B12), phytonutrients (including phycocyanin), selenium, zinc, copper, manganese, iron (22 times the amount of spinach), vitamin E and gamma-linolenic acid (an omega-6 fatty acid).

PIÑA COLADA MILK

INGREDIENTS:

Use the *Coconut Milk* recipe above
(4 CUPS), then add:

1 ½ CUPS
Fresh Pineapple
(or 1 cup pineapple juice)

PREPARATION:

01. Add Coconut Milk and pineapple, starting with half the pineapple the recipe calls for (¾ cup) to a blender and blend for 2 minutes. Taste and continue to add pineapple until you reach the desired flavor. Fresh produce varies significantly, so I usually start with ¾ - 1 cup of fresh pineapple and add from there until I reach my desired sweet and piña coladaness!

02. Blend and refrigerate immediately until ready to use.

OAT MILK

INGREDIENTS:

1 CUP
Rolled Oats (gluten-free)

4 CUPS
Ice Cold Water
(use 3 ½ cups for a creamier oat milk)

⅛ TSP
Himalayan Salt

2 LARGE
Medjool Dates, pitted

1 TSP
Pure Vanilla Extract

1 TBSP
Coconut Oil
OPTIONAL: you'll want to add an oil if you plan to heat your oat milk.

PREPARATION:

01. Combine all of the ingredients in a high speed blender and blend for approximately 20 seconds, or until the mixture seems well combined. It doesn't have to be 100% pulverized. In fact, over-blending can make the oat milk slimy in texture. The ice cold water also helps to make sure your oat milk isn't slimy.

02. Carefully strain the mixture through a nut milk bag or a sieve and discard the pulp (unless you plan to reuse the pulp for any reason). I like to strain first through a sieve, then a nut milk bag. Unlike nut milk, you do not want to squeeze anything through the nut milk bag. This will result in a slimy oat milk. Let what passes, pass.

03. Transfer to a sealed container and refrigerate. Will keep in the refrigerator up to 5 days (sometimes more). Shake well before using.

GOLDEN MILK

INGREDIENTS:

Use the *Oat Milk* recipe above (**4 CUPS**), then add:

7 LARGE
Medjool Dates, pitted

½ TSP + ⅛ TSP
Turmeric Juice

¼ TSP
Cardamom

1 PINCH
Black Pepper

PREPARATION:

01. Add 4 cups of prepared Oat Milk and dates to a high speed blender and blend until dates are thoroughly blended. Be careful not to overblend, as your oat milk will get slimy. Add the remaining ingredients and blend just until combined, about 10 seconds. This recipe can also be made with Sprouted Vanilla Almond Milk or Hemp Milk.

NOTE:
Did you know turmeric is one of the best anti-inflammatory spices on the planet? You should also know that when you add just a pinch of black pepper to any recipe with turmeric (including the Golden Milk recipe above), it increases the anti-inflammatory benefits! Plus, you get increased absorption and magnified effects when these two spices are combined.

HEMP MILK

INGREDIENTS:

1 CUP
Raw Hemp Seeds

4 CUPS
Water
(use 3 cups for a creamier milk)

1 PINCH
Himalayan Salt

4 LARGE
Medjool Dates, pitted

1 TSP
Pure Vanilla Extract

PREPARATION:

01. Combine all of the ingredients in a high speed blender and blend until the raw hemp seeds are completely broken down (approximately 1-2 minutes). Carefully strain the mixture through a nut milk bag and discard the pulp.

    <u>NOTE</u>:
    You can store the pulp for a few days in the fridge and add it to smoothies, baking, oatmeal, or anything else, really.

02. Transfer to a sealed container and refrigerate. Will keep in the refrigerator up to 5 days (sometimes more). Shake well before using.

    <u>OPTIONAL</u>:
    I love adding a tablespoon or two of coconut butter to this recipe! I think it brings a balanced flavor and tones down the intensity of the hemp.

CHOCOLATE HEMP MILK

INGREDIENTS:

Use the *Hemp Milk* recipe above
(4 CUPS), then add:

6 LARGE
Medjool Dates, pitted

5 TBSP
Raw Cacao Powder

¼ TSP
Cinnamon

1 PINCH
Himalayan Salt

PREPARATION:

01. Add all ingredients to a high speed blender and blend for about 2 minutes or until dates are thoroughly blended. Refrigerate or enjoy immediately. You can add more dates depending on how sweet you want your milk.

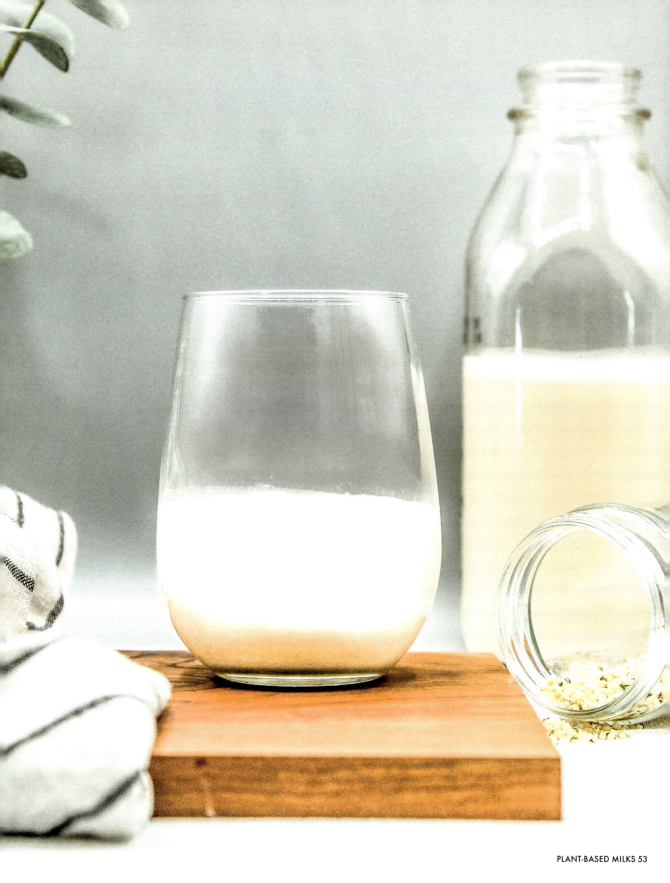

CHAPTER 5

54 ELIXIRS / LATTES

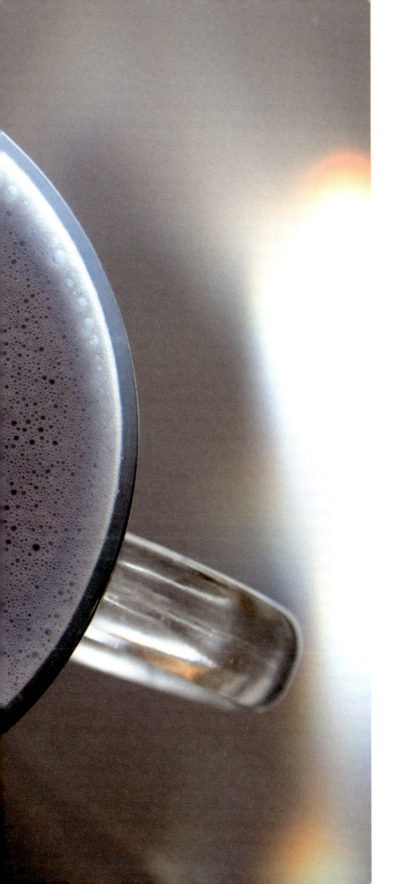

ELIXIRS & LATTÉS

Nothing makes me happier than a nice warm latté or a hot elixir in hand, especially on those cold fall and winter days (and nights). Lattés and elixirs can be so great for you when they are loaded with homemade and organic ingredients and are crafted to be healing and delicious. Unfortunately, it's quite rare to find truly healthy lattés at your local coffee shop. We have an extensive and healthy latté and elixir menu at Choice, but if you are looking to expand your repertoire of homemade elixirs and lattés, then get excited because this chapter is for you!

I was never much of a coffee drinker prior to Choice. In fact, I had never even had a sip of coffee before testing the recipe for our cold-pressed coffee (I know, shocker, right?). When gearing up to open Choice, I realized there was a need for people to have a healthier way to caffeinate. I learned a lot about cold-pressed coffee, including the fact that it can be up to 75% less acidic than traditional coffee when prepared this way. This allows you to reap the benefits (antioxidants) in the coffee without an exorbitant amount of acidity (which can create excess inflammation, a big no-no for your health).

Here are some of my favorite recipes, which I hope you'll enjoy as well!

COLD-PRESSED COFFEE

INGREDIENTS:

1 *CUP*
Organic Coffee Grounds

4 *CUPS*
Filtered Water

PREPARATION:

01. Soak for a minimum of 8 hours, maximum of 16 hours (8 hours will give you a lighter coffee flavor while 12-16 hours will give you a nice deep coffee flavor).

02. Press through a nut milk bag with a bowl beneath to catch the Cold-Pressed Coffee. Discard grounds (option to toss the Cold-Pressed Coffee grounds in your garden or find another creative use).

03. Store in an airtight container and refrigerate immediately. This will store for up to 2 weeks.

COLD-PRESSED COFFEE LATTÉ

Use your favorite plant-based milk recipe from chapter 4 (I prefer the Sprouted Vanilla Almond Milk or the Oat Milk for this one).

INGREDIENTS:

8 *OZ.*
Cold-Pressed Coffee

8 *OZ.*
Plant-Based Milk

3 *LARGE*
Medjool Dates, pitted
(more if you like it extra sweet)

1 *PINCH*
Cinnamon *(OPTIONAL)*

PREPARATION: *(16OZ.)*

01. Place all ingredients in a high speed blender and blend for approximately 1 minute until the dates are fully blended in. Portion between two cups and enjoy. You can enjoy this as is or pour over ice for an iced coffee experience.

NOTE:

Don't let this small serving size fool you. Cold-Pressed Coffee is way more potent than traditional coffee! You only need half a cup of cold-pressed to caffeinate you as much as a full cup of traditional coffee would. That being said, Cold-Pressed Coffee is up to 75% less acidic than traditional coffee. The antioxidant properties of coffee are always being touted as a huge health benefit to drinking that daily cup of Joe and while that's true, with all the acidity, it's hard to reap those benefits.

Trust me, this is not your average coffee - it's better!

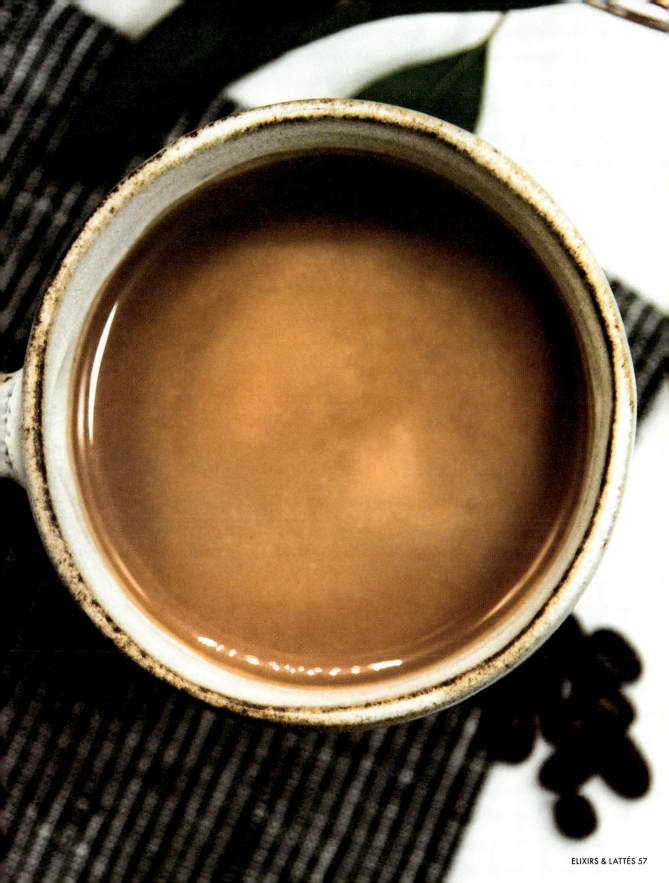

GOLDEN LATTÉ

This Golden Latté is a delicious and easy way to get more of one of the world's most powerful anti-inflammatory foods into your daily life. It's boosted with black pepper, which unlocks turmeric's bioavailability. This latté is so simple and yet, so delicious. Especially when made with homemade almond milk. Sweetening this latté with coconut sugar, gives it a nice healthy sweet flavor. The best part is the recipe only takes about 5 minutes to make!

INGREDIENTS:

8 OZ
Sprouted Vanilla Almond Milk

½ TSP
Turmeric Powder

1 PINCH
Black Pepper

¼ TSP
Cardamom Powder

2 TSP
Coconut Sugar

¼ TSP
Ginger

PREPARATION:

01. Place the Sprouted Vanilla Almond Milk and spices in a small pot and bring to a light boil. Pour into your favorite mug and enjoy immediately.

NOTE:
If you have a frother, use it! It adds to the fun of this at-home latté.

CHAGA LATTÉ

My take on a traditional hot cocoa - basically a super potent medicinal hot chocolate!

Often referred to as the "King of the Mushrooms," Chaga is a known adaptogen which basically means that it adapts to the body and provides it with what it needs. Loaded with melanin and vitamin D, this magic mushroom protects your skin and boosts your health. Chaga is one of the highest alkaline foods on the planet, helping balance your body's pH. It is also extremely high in antioxidants, which help fight free radicals that can cause cell damage.

This Chaga Latté is a delicious and nutritious way to reap the many benefits of this adaptogenic medicinal mushroom.

INGREDIENTS:

1 CUP
Oat Milk or Sprouted Vanilla Almond Milk

1 TBSP
Cacao

1 TSP
Chaga Mushroom Powder

2 TSP
Coconut Sugar

1 TSP
Lucuma

⅛ TSP
Cinnamon

1 PINCH
Himalayan Salt

PREPARATION:

01. Add all ingredients to a blender and blend on high for 20-30 seconds.

02. Place into a tea pot or small pot and heat (without boiling).

03. Pour into your favorite mug and enjoy immediately.

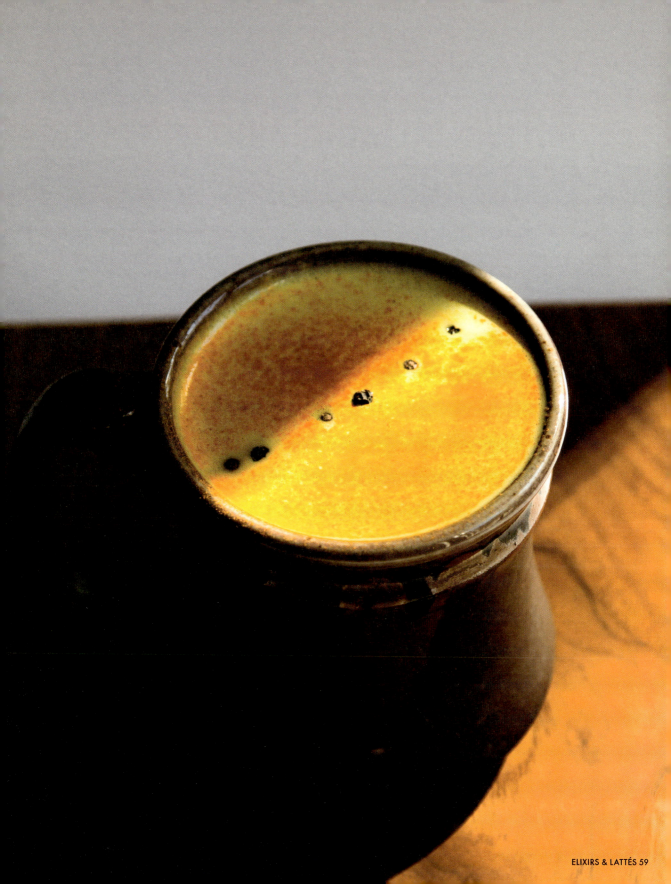

ACTIVATED CHARCOAL LEMONADE

I'm sure you've seen charcoal beverages including lemonades, cocktails and more, hitting the shelves at all your favorite juice shops and hipster bars and there is certainly a good reason for this. Activated charcoal alleviates gas and bloating, rids the body of artificial sugars and chemicals, and helps with digestion. It also happens to be an incredible hangover cure. Not that I am endorsing the over consumption of alcohol, but if you find yourself hurting after partying a little too hard, activated charcoal can have you feeling better in no time.

There are a couple of things to consider when diving into the charcoal waters. First, make sure you find coconut activated charcoal that is ultra fine and food grade! Second, don't overdo it! Activated charcoal can interfere with the absorption of medication, as well as some vitamins. That being said, this is NOT an everyday drink. Once a week or a couple of times a month is more than enough to make sure you're not overdoing the detoxifying effects of charcoal. Lemon is also very alkalizing, despite it's acidic flavor.

INGREDIENTS:

1/4 CUP
Lemon Juice

2 CUPS
Water

2 TBSP
Monk Fruit

1 TSP
Activated Charcoal

PREPARATION:

01. Add lemon to water then whisk in the activated charcoal and monk fruit, until the powders are mixed thoroughly. Place in the fridge for a few hours to chill. I love to serve this over ice.

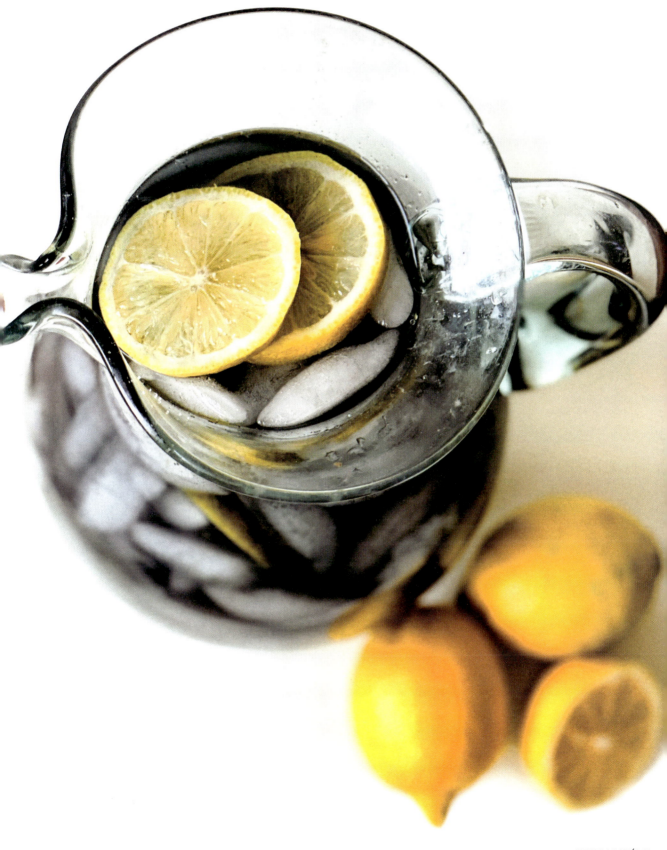

IMMUNITY TEA

This healing elixir is my absolute favorite when I'm feeling under the weather or when I've been around others who haven't been feeling well. Of course, I'm always taking my Immunity Shots at Choice and I swear by them. But when I need something more, this always does the trick for me!

Ginger is filled with immune-boosting benefits, making it one of my favorite go-to ingredients. First off, ginger is antibacterial so it helps support the immune system and it can help to prevent nausea and soothe an upset stomach. According to Ayurveda, ginger warms the body and helps to break down the accumulation of toxins in the organs, particularly in the lungs and sinuses. Ginger helps to cleanse the lymphatic system, which is our body's sewage system. By opening up these lymphatic channels and keeping things clean, ginger prevents the accumulation of the toxins that make you susceptible to infections, especially in the respiratory system. It doesn't take long to see the benefits of ginger when you have a sore throat or a cold. Ginger is a must-have food during cold and flu season.

Lemons contain lots of antioxidants and vitamin C. Foods that are high in vitamin C and other antioxidants help strengthen the immune system against the germs that cause colds and the flu. Lemons also help with the acid/alkaline balance in the body. As such, incorporating lemon into your diet regularly may make your body less susceptible to illnesses.

Cloves boost immune system function, aid in treating colds, are anti-inflammatory and antibacterial. Cloves have been shown to help fight infections, relieve digestive problems and arthritis pain.

Cinnamon is known to boost the immune system and may help ward off colds and the flu thanks to its antibacterial and antimicrobial properties and antioxidant activities.

Cardamom is considered the "Queen of Spices" with an impressive list of exceptional wellness perks! Ayurvedic medicine has recognized the merits of the spice for over 5,000 years, prescribing it for everything from digestive disorders to infectious illnesses.

INGREDIENTS:

¾ CUP
Lemon Juice

3 ½ CUPS
Water

¼ CUP
Coconut Nectar

2 IN.
Fresh Ginger,
unpeeled and coarsely chopped

4
Cloves

1
Cardamom Pod

1
Cinnamon Stick

PREPARATION:

01. In a medium saucepan combine lemon juice, water, coconut nectar, ginger, and spices. Bring to a simmer, stirring until nectar is dissolved. Remove from heat and cover, allowing to steep for 15 minutes.

02. Strain and serve immediately.

(OPTION:)
Turn into immunity lemonade by refrigerating until chilled through. Serve over ice.

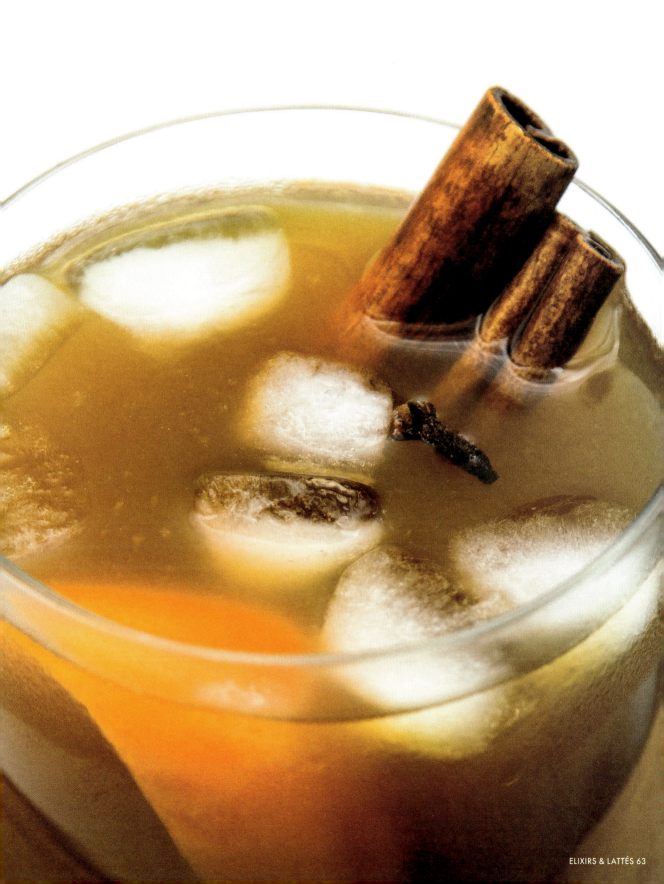

ELIXIRS & LATTÉS 63

MUSHROOM COFFEE LATTÉ

This is the perfect blend of sweet and creamy coffee with a boost of healing mushrooms to healthify your morning routine. And don't worry, even if you're not a fan of the fungi, you will love this drink (you can't even taste the mushy's)! If you're a religious coffee drinker, boosting your coffee with superfoods is a great way to increase your intake of healing plants (plus lower the acidity) and gain all the benefits.

INGREDIENTS:

½ CUP
Oat Milk or Sprouted Vanilla Almond Milk

½ CUP
Cold-Pressed Coffee

1 TSP
Chaga Mushroom Powder

1 TSP
Reishi Mushroom Powder

1 TBSP
Coconut Sugar

1 TSP
Lucuma

⅛ TSP
Cinnamon

1 PINCH
Himalayan Salt

PREPARATION:

01. In a small saucepan, warm the plant-based milk and Cold-Pressed Coffee, being careful not to boil.

02. Add warmed milk and coffee along with the remaining ingredients, to a high powered blender and blend for 30 seconds.

03. Pour and drink immediately.

ICED MATCHA LATTÉ

If the taste of a yummy Iced Matcha Latté isn't enough to get you psyched about drinking matcha, here are few additional reasons.

Matcha is very high in antioxidants and is known for increasing energy while providing a calming effect, unlike its other caffeinated counterparts. Matcha also has fat burning effects due to a compound called EGCG (epigallocatechin gallate), a polyphenol, which has been shown to boost metabolism and stop the growth of fat cells. A few more benefits of matcha include increased brain power, focus and mental clarity due to L-Theanine, which is found in green tea. It's also well documented for promoting beautiful skin by reducing inflammation and free radicals, those nasty things that can accelerate skin aging, yuck!

INGREDIENTS:

1 TSP
Matcha Green Tea Powder

1 TBSP
Hot Water

1 OZ (2 TBSP)
Water, room temperature

2 TSP
Monk Fruit

1/4 TSP
Reishi Powder

6 OZ
Sprouted Vanilla Almond Milk

1/2 TSP
Liquid Chlorophyll

3/4 CUP
Ice

EQUIPMENT NEEDED:

Bamboo Whisk. *Not absolutely necessary, but creates a much smoother and frothier drink than a regular whisk.*

TIP:
In a pinch, use a blender.

PREPARATION:

01. Mix the matcha green tea powder with the hot water in a bowl until well combined.

02. Add the 2 Tbsp of room temp. water and whisk again until well combined.

03. Next, add in the monk fruit and reishi powder and whisk well.

04. Place some ice cubes in a glass and add the Sprouted Vanilla Almond Milk.

05. Next, add the matcha mixture and stir.

06. Finally, add your liquid chlorophyll and stir. If you like your matcha on the sweeter side, you can add an additional 1 tsp of monk fruit or swap monk fruit for 2 tsp of coconut sugar.

MAJIK LAVENDER LATTÉ

This Majik Lavender Latté is both delicious and healing. Lavender has a calming effect, which makes it an ideal addition to an evening latté, and the perfect way to relax away stress and anxiety, any time of day. Blue Majik adds protein, omega-3s, antioxidants, B vitamins and helps to nourish your body at a cellular level.

INGREDIENTS:

1 ½ CUPS
Sprouted Vanilla Almond Milk

2 LARGE
Medjool Dates, pitted

¼ TSP
E3Live Blue Majik

½ TSP
Lavender Flowers
(can be purchased online or in some health food stores)

½ TSP
Lucuma

PREPARATION:

01. In a small saucepan, warm the Sprouted Vanilla Almond Milk, taking care not to boil.

02. Add warmed Sprouted Vanilla Almond Milk and all remaining ingredients to a high powered blender and blend for 30 seconds, or until dates are thoroughly blended.

03. Pour and drink immediately.

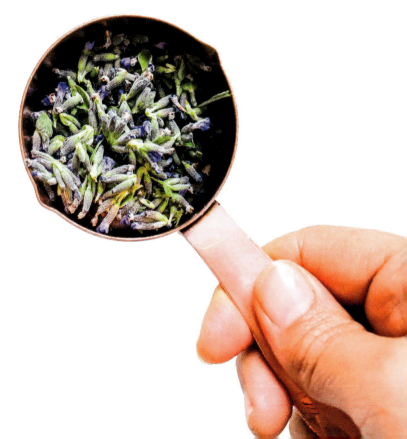

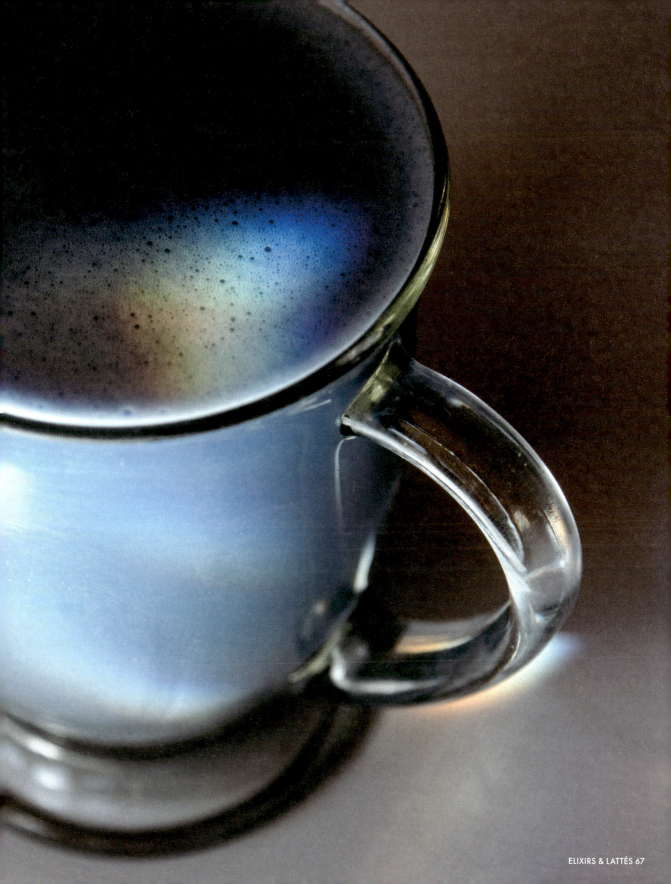

BEETROOT ROSE CARDAMOM LATTÉ

Beets are known to lower blood pressure, boost endurance and stamina, promote weight loss, prevent anemia, are great for digestion, promote liver detoxification, are known to improve heart health and increase energy.

Pink rose petal powder cools and soothes the body, balances vata and pitta (Ayurveda), supports the nervous system, is anti-aging and contains naturally uplifting properties that promote positive feelings and help to balance your mood.

Cardamom is great for oral health, is also heart healthy, may lower blood pressure levels and is known to help fight depression.

Monk fruit contains compounds that, when extracted, are natural sweeteners 300–400 times the sweetness of cane sugar without the calories and has zero effect on blood sugar. Sound too good to be true? It's not! This fruit has been used as a sweetener for centuries and it's only recently become popular in the U.S. Along with its magical sweetening powers, monk fruit has long been regarded as the "longevity fruit" thanks to its high antioxidant levels. Throughout history, it was also used medicinally as a cough remedy and for help with other respiratory ailments. It was also utilized for constipation, as a treatment for diabetes, and as a way to clear heat from the body caused by both internal and external sources.

INGREDIENTS:

1 1/2 CUPS
Oat Milk or Sprouted Vanilla Almond Milk

1/2 TSP
Beetroot Powder

1/4 TSP
Pink Rose Petal Powder

1/4 TSP
Cardamom

1 TBSP
Monk Fruit

PREPARATION:

01. In a small saucepan, warm the Sprouted Vanilla Almond Milk, taking care not to boil.

02. Add warmed Oat Milk or Sprouted Vanilla Almond Milk and all remaining ingredients to a high powered blender and blend for 30 seconds.

03. Pour and drink immediately.

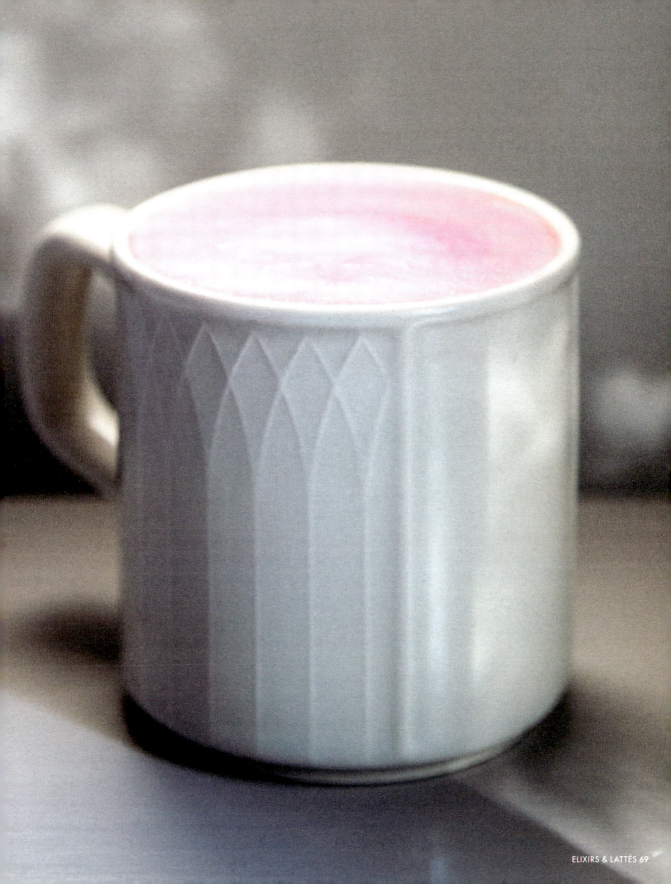

PUMPKIN SPICED FRAPPÉ

One of my favorite seasons is pumpkin season - I am obsessed with all things pumpkin! This Pumpkin Spiced Frappé is perfect for our San Diego fall months. With our beautiful warm weather, I find myself craving pumpkin smoothies and iced frappés regularly and this frappé always satisfies my pumpkin cravings!

INGREDIENTS:

1 CUP
Sprouted Vanilla Almond Milk

1/2 CUP
Cold-Pressed Coffee

2 TBSP
Pumpkin Purée

2 LARGE
Medjool Dates, pitted

1 1/2 TSP
Pumpkin Spice
(SEE RECIPE TO THE RIGHT)

1/8 TSP
Cinnamon

3/4 CUP
Ice

3 TBSP
Coconut Whipped Cream
(OPTIONAL: RECIPE ON PG. 210)

PREPARATION:

01. Add all ingredients, except ice, to a high powered blender and blend for 30 seconds, or until the dates are thoroughly blended.

02. Add ice and blend until you get a frappé consistency.

03. Top with Coconut Whipped Cream and enjoy immediately.

PUMPKIN SPICE

INGREDIENTS:

3 TBSP
Ground Cinnamon

4 TSP
Ground Ginger

1/2 TSP
Ground Nutmeg

1/4 TSP
Ground Clove

1/8 TSP
Allspice

1/4 TSP
Ground Black Pepper

1/4 TSP
Ground Cardamom

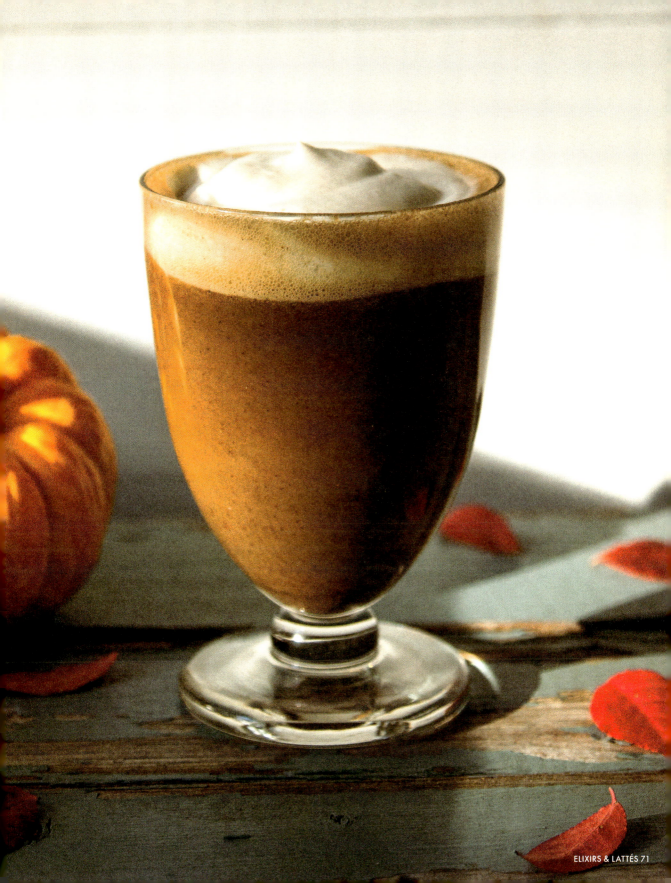

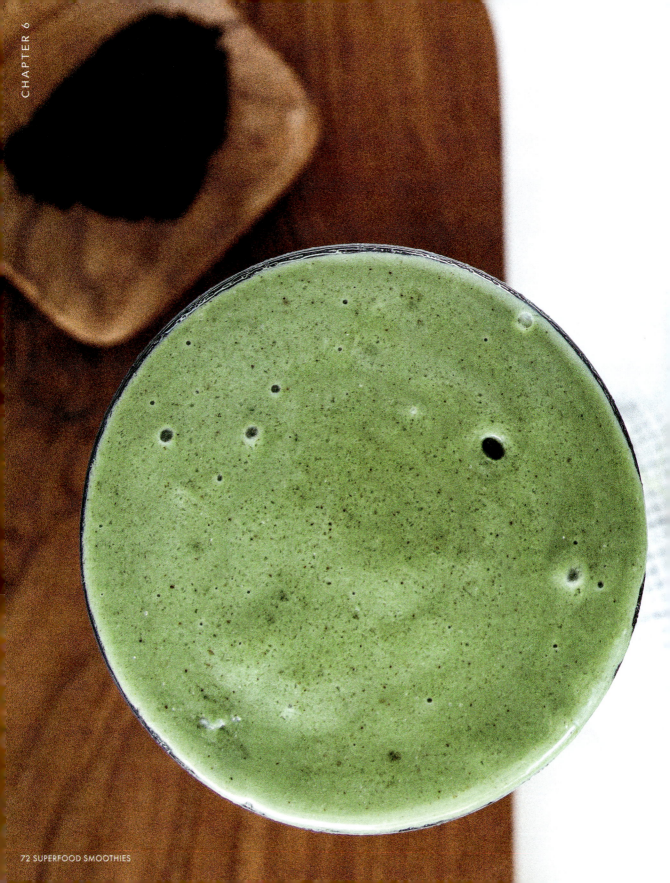

SUPERFOOD SMOOTHIES

Smoothies, specifically superfood smoothies, are a delicious way to boost your nutrition intake without too much effort. Toss a few things in a blender and voila! I've been drinking a smoothie for breakfast every single day for more than a decade. I find it helps me with maintaining a healthy lifestyle. I believe that what you eat for breakfast really does set the stage for the rest of your day. Having a superfood smoothie for breakfast will help you to feel great in your body. You'll feel more energized and you'll be more likely to stick to better choices throughout the day! Kicking the day off with a superfood smoothie that's loaded with protein, fiber, tons of vitamins and minerals—that's both filling and nutritious—is definitely the right choice in my book.

Smoothie Making DOS & DON'TS

Maybe you're already an expert smoothie maker or maybe this is your first go at making a homemade superfood smoothie. Either way, there are a few things to consider (or remember).

NOT ALL BLENDERS ARE CREATED EQUALLY
Sad, but true! We use Vitamix blenders at Choice because they do the best job at blending, in my experience. That being said, you can still make an awesome smoothie with just about any blender. However, I recommend using a high powered blender to get the best blend (which makes for the smoothest consistency and yummiest smoothies).

PRE-BLEND
This is a very important step in making the perfect smoothie. It's tempting to toss all your ingredients in at the same time, but for the perfect flavor and consistency, you want to pre-blend some of your ingredients. You're always going to pre-blend your plant-based milk, with your powders (protein, superfoods, etc.), dates (or whatever you're using to sweeten your smoothie), nut butters, nuts, seeds and produce. See *blending order* below for more details.

BLENDING ORDER
This is more important than most realize. As mentioned above, you want to follow a specific order to get the perfect consistency and flavor.

HERE'S THE ORDER

1st. BLEND: Plant-based milk, powders, nut butters, fresh produce (such as spinach, oranges, kale, etc.), sweeteners (this is especially important when using whole dates to sweeten your smoothies because the last thing you want are pieces of date chunks in your finished smoothie).

2nd. BLEND: This is when you'll toss in your frozen goodies. The only exception to this rule is acaí. Acaí packs are treated like fresh produce and tossed into the first blend. Aside from acaí, any frozen fruit will get tossed in on the second blend, including ice.

3rd. BLEND: The third blend isn't going to apply to every smoothie, just the smoothies that you want to add a little cacao crunch to or if you prefer ingredients like hemp seeds to add some texture instead of being fully blended.

BLEND TIME
Your first blend is always going to be high speed for 60 seconds (this may be longer if you aren't working with a high powered blender, in which case, make sure you blend until you don't see any big pieces flying around in the blender). You want to be sure that all items are fully pulverized in this step to save you from over blending after your second blend (if there are still pieces of date, nuts, seeds, etc.).

Your second blend can vary based on the recipe and blender you are using. That being said, it's important to start with a shorter time like 30 seconds. Check your smoothie and if it's not fully blended or if it's too thick, put it on for another 30 seconds at high speed. You can always blend more, but you can't fix an over blended smoothie.

DOS

01. **Get creative.** Smoothies are a great way to get creative with healthy goodies, and superfoods. Try adding reishi mushrooms, maca, baobab or any other amazing superfoods that intrigue your senses. Just start with a small amount and go from there!

02. **Have fun.** The great thing about smoothies is that they are easy to whip up. So have fun with it.

03. **Toss in those leafy greens.** You won't taste them so it's any easy way to increase your daily veggie intake, especially when you're making smoothies for your kiddos.

04. **Use your plant-based milks as the base for your smoothies for the ultimate nutritional value.**

05. **Get yourself a good reusable straw.** If you're anything like me, you have to drink a smoothie from a straw. So invest in a good reusable straw so you can get the full experience at home.

DON'TS

01. **Ripe bananas = slimy smoothies.** Always slice and freeze your bananas in advance for creamy, thick, delicious smoothies.

02. **Never add coconut butter after you've already added your frozens.** It needs to be pre-blended. You can mess up on almost any nut butter and get away with tossing it in after the fact, without the risk of over blending. This is not true of coconut butter. It needs to be emulsified in the first blend otherwise, it will clump up on you. So unless you like little hard clumps of coconut butter, never add this after you've blended your frozen ingredients. Always pre-blend!

03. **Don't over blend!** I discussed this above, but it's worth mentioning again. The perfect smoothie is thick, cold and delicious. Runny smoothies are a no-no in the Choice world. So make sure you're paying attention to your blend time!

04. **Don't save for later.** Smoothies are meant to be enjoyed immediately. Don't get tempted to double batch your smoothie so you can enjoy a hassle free smoothie tomorrow! Blend, pour and drink! Plus, this guarantees maximum nutrition.

Okay, so now that we've established some ground rules for creating epic smoothies, here are some of my favorite recipes for you to try at home!

CONTROL CRAVINGS
Keeps You Feeling Full
Antioxidants
IMMUNITY
Improved Skin
DETOXING
Brain Power
ELEVATED MOODS
Bone Health

HORMONE BALANCING

Increased Intake of Fruits & Veggies

QUICK AND EASY

Easy Way to BOOST Kids' Nutrition Intake

Improved digestion

BEAUTY

HEALTHY BRAIN FUNCTION

FIGHTS DEPRESSION

CHOCOLATE PEANUT BUTTER CUP

Why you should drink it: High in protein, calcium, magnesium, increases energy, mood enhancing, high in antioxidants and hormone balancing.

It's like dessert for breakfast! One of my favorite childhood treats was a chocolate peanut butter cup. This smoothie is reminiscent of just that. But of course, it's a much healthier version. That being said, your taste buds won't be disappointed.

INGREDIENTS:

1 CUP
Frozen Banana

1 CUP
Ice

2 LARGE
Medjool Dates, pitted

1 CUP
Sprouted Vanilla Almond Milk

1 TBSP
Peanut Butter

1 TBSP
Choice Superfood Protein
(available in stores or online)

1 ½ TBSP
Cacao Powder

PREPARATION:

01. Pre-blend the Sprouted Vanilla Almond Milk, dates, Choice Superfood Protein, cacao powder and peanut butter.

02. Then toss in your frozen banana and ice. Blend until thick, smooth and creamy, then enjoy!

BONUS:
A fun way to boost your vitamin intake here without changing the flavor profile, is by adding a handful of spinach. Spinach is loaded with magnesium, potassium, zinc, iron, calcium, vitamin K and vitamin C to name a few. Don't forget to pre-blend your spinach if you are going to add it (see blending order on pg. 74).

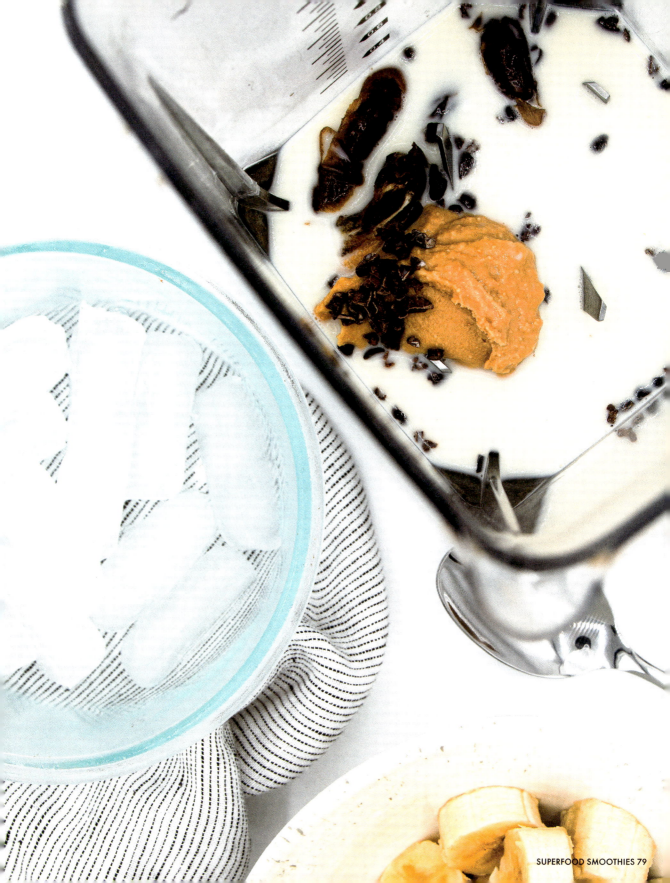

BLUE HERO

Why you should drink it: This smoothie is delicious and teeming with nutrition. It's sweetened naturally with whole dates, and contains lots of protein from the hemp, protein powder and Blue Majik. The hemp is also a great source of iron, omega-3s and fiber. Oh, and it has a brilliant blue hue, which makes it that much more fun to drink! It also packs a nutritional punch by helping to improve recovery time from workouts, increase brain function and nourish your body on a cellular level.

If the color of this smoothie alone doesn't make you want to guzzle this thing down, then the flavor and bountiful nutrients certainly will!

INGREDIENTS:

1 CUP
Frozen Banana

1 CUP
Ice

2 LARGE
Medjool Dates, pitted

1 CUP
Sprouted Vanilla Almond Milk

1 TBSP
Hemp Seeds

1 TBSP
Choice Superfood Protein
(available in stores or online)

1 TSP
E3live Blue Majik

PREPARATION:

01. Pre-blend the Sprouted Vanilla Almond Milk, dates, Choice Superfood Protein, Blue Majik, and hemp seeds.

02. Then toss in your frozen banana and ice. Blend until thick, smooth and creamy, then enjoy!

NOTE:

Don't be fooled by cheap imitations! At Choice, we are always committed to using the highest quality ingredients, so we use E3Live Blue Majik, and you should too. E3live brought the world Blue Majik—a certified organic 100% Phycocyanin extract.

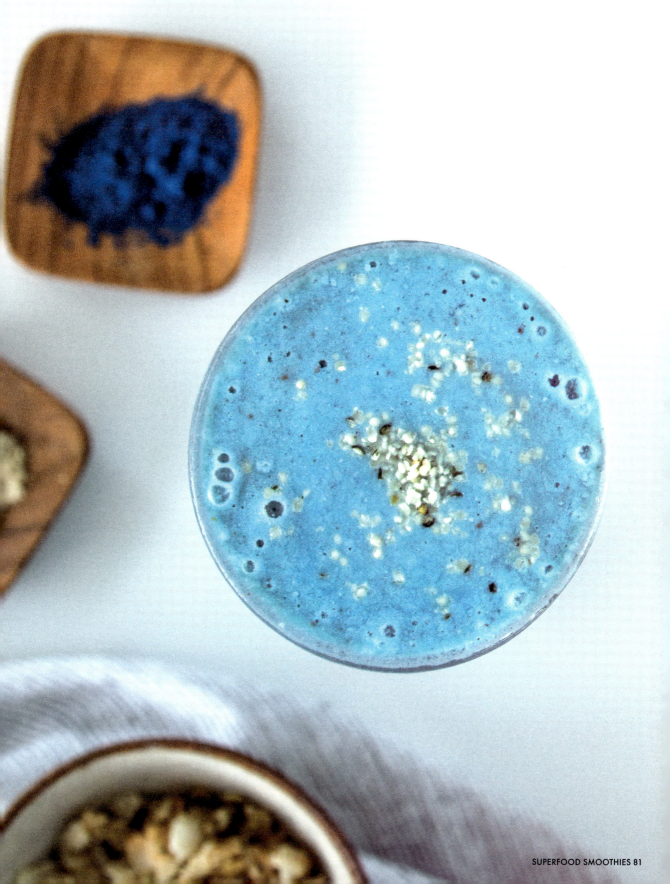

CHOCOLATE STRAWBERRY

Why you should drink it: Protein, fiber, immune boosting, alkalizing, high in vitamin C, manganese potassium and folate.

This smoothie seriously tastes like a chocolate covered strawberry! Who doesn't love chocolate covered strawberries? It's also full of nutrition. Win win!

INGREDIENTS:

1 CUP
Frozen Banana

1 CUP
Frozen Strawberries

1 CUP
Sprouted Vanilla Almond Milk

2 LARGE
Medjool Dates, pitted

1 TBSP
Choice Superfood Protein
(available online or in stores)

1 TBSP
Cacao Nibs

PREPARATION:

01. Pre-blend the Sprouted Vanilla Almond Milk, dates and Choice Superfood Protein.

02. Toss in the frozen banana and strawberries. Blend until thick, smooth and creamy.

03. Add the cacao nibs and blend on high for 4 seconds, then enjoy!

SUGGESTIONS:

Add a handful of spinach or ½ tsp E3live Blue Majik for an additional boost of nutrition, or try adding 1 Tbsp of peanut butter for extra protein and a fun twist!

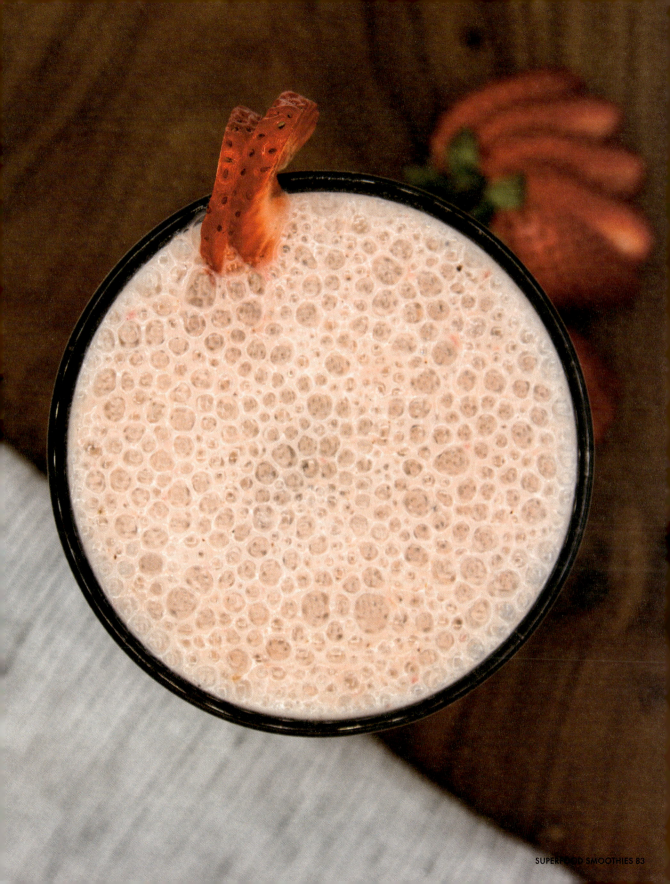

JAVA CHIP

Why you should drink it: Protein, increased energy, mood enhancing, hormone balancing, antioxidants, calcium and magnesium.

Coffee ice cream is one of my all time favorites, so you won't be surprised to learn this is one of my favorite smoothies. It literally tastes just like coffee ice cream, only it's sweetened naturally with whole fruit and it's super low in acidity because it's made with plant-based milk and Cold-Pressed Coffee.

INGREDIENTS:

1 CUP
Frozen Banana

1 CUP
Ice

½ CUP
Sprouted Vanilla Almond Milk
(or Oat Milk)

½ CUP
Cold-Pressed Coffee

2 LARGE
Medjool Dates, pitted

1 TBSP
Choice Superfood Protein
(available in stores or online)

1 TBSP
Coconut Butter

1 TBSP
Cacao Nibs

1 TSP
Maca Powder

PREPARATION:

01. Pre-blend the Sprouted Vanilla Almond Milk, Cold-Pressed Coffee, dates, Choice Superfood Protein, maca and coconut butter.

02. Toss in the frozen banana and ice. Blend until thick, smooth and creamy

03. Add the cacao nibs and blend on high for 4 seconds. Enjoy immediately!

<u>SUGGESTIONS</u>:
Swap coconut butter for peanut butter for a delicious peanut butter twist!

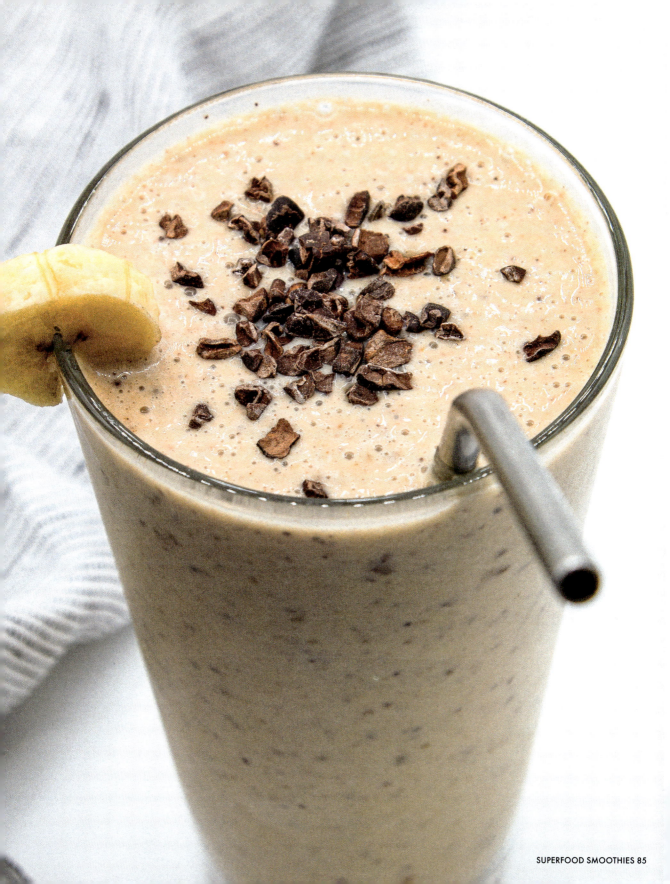

SALTED CARAMEL

Why you should drink it: High in protein, fiber, immune boosting, high mineral content, antifungal, omega-3s.

Mesquite is highly underrated in the superfood world. This is not the same part of the mesquite that gives you that smokey BBQ flavor. This is actually the edible pod from the plant! It's loaded with nutrition and it just so happens to have a natural caramel flavor, making it a perfect addition to this Salted Caramel smoothie.

INGREDIENTS:

1 TBSP
Coconut Caramel Sauce
(more if desired - recipe on pg. 210)

1 CUP
Frozen Banana

1 CUP
Ice

1 CUP
Sprouted Vanilla Almond Milk
(or Oat Milk)

2 LARGE
Medjool Dates, pitted

1 TBSP
Choice Superfood Protein
(available online or in stores)

¼ TSP
Himalayan Salt

1 ½ TBSP
Mesquite Powder

1 TBSP
Almond Butter

PREPARATION:

01. Pre-blend the Sprouted Vanilla Almond Milk, dates, Choice Superfood Protein, mesquite, Himalayan salt and almond butter.

02. Toss in the frozen banana and ice. Blend until thick, smooth and creamy.

03. Drizzle the Coconut Caramel Sauce all around a cup and on top of your smoothie, then enjoy!

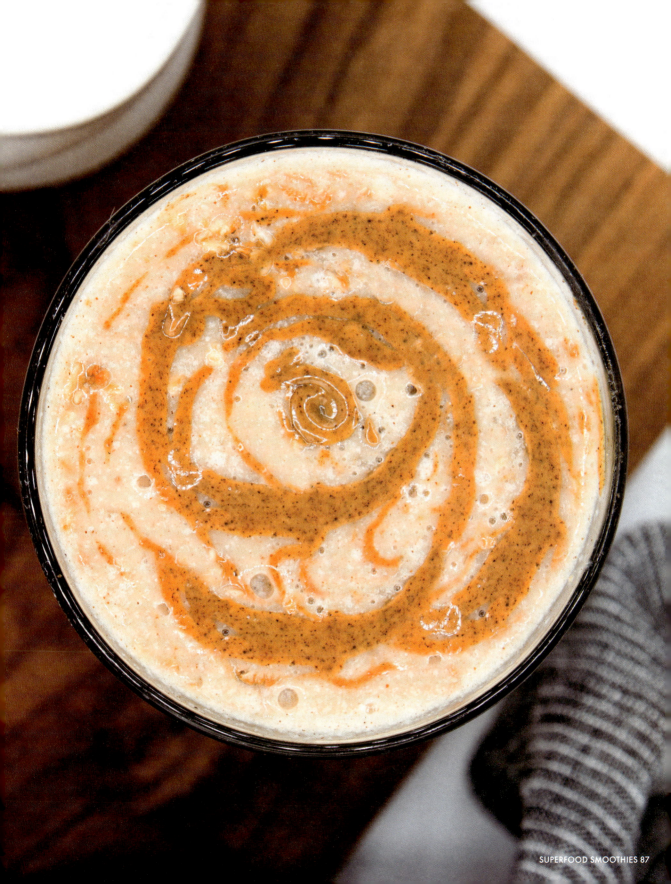

GREEN MACHINE

Why you should drink it: High in protein, fiber, immune boosting, energizing, high mineral content, omega-3s, alkalizing, anti-inflammatory.

Don't let all the greens in this smoothie deter you. It tastes like a creamy vanilla shake even though it's loaded with all sorts of amazingness. Don't just take my word for it, give it a try!

INGREDIENTS:

1 CUP
Frozen Banana

1 CUP
Ice

1 CUP
Sprouted Vanilla Almond Milk
(or Oat Milk)

2 LARGE
Medjool Dates, pitted

1 TBSP
Choice Superfood Protein
(available online or in stores)

1 TSP
Spirulina

½ CUP
Spinach (about a handful)

1 TBSP
Almond Butter

PREPARATION:

01. Pre-blend the Sprouted Vanilla Almond Milk, dates, Choice Superfood Protein, spirulina, almond butter and spinach.

02. Then toss in your frozen banana and ice. Blend until thick, smooth and creamy, then enjoy!

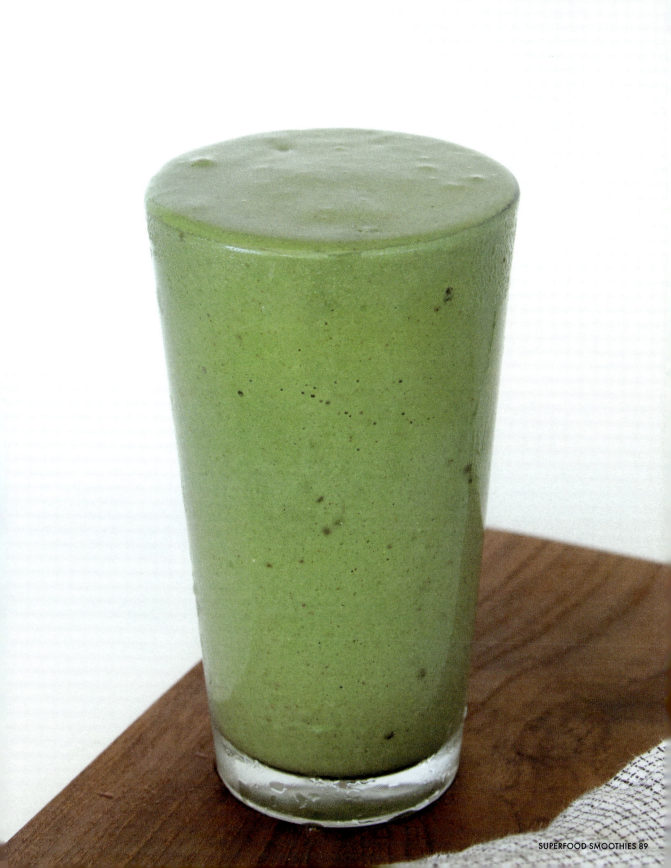

CHAPTER 7

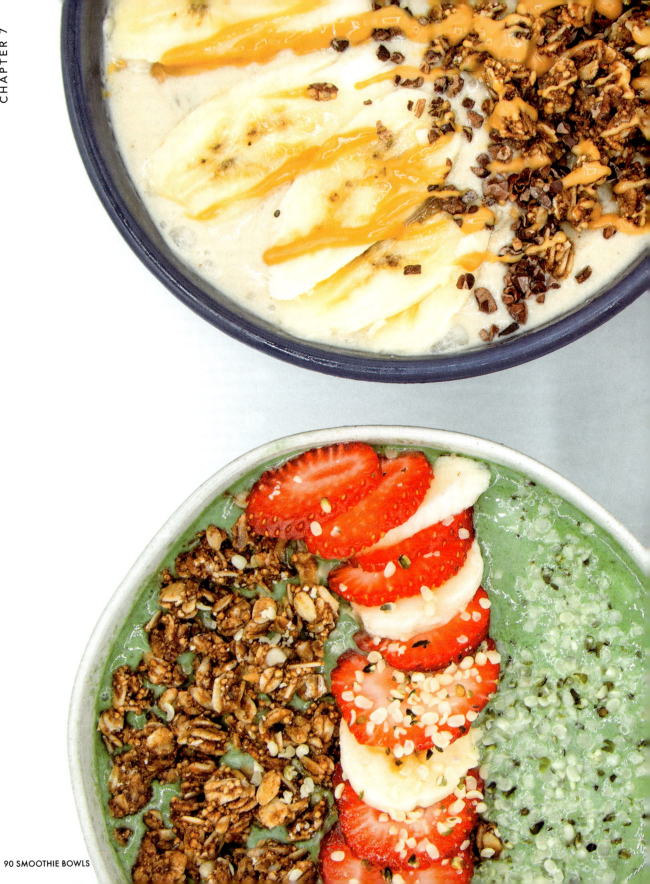

90 SMOOTHIE BOWLS

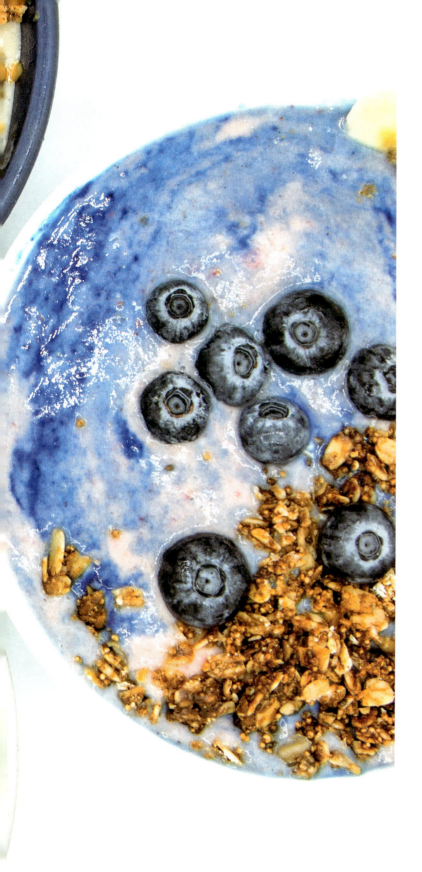

SMOOTHIE BOWLS

A smoothie bowl is basically a thicker smoothie served in a bowl! It's a great option when you're really hungry and are craving something a little more substantial than a smoothie. It's also a great substitute for ice cream, which we know is full of processed sugar amongst other unnecessary and unhealthy ingredients. I remember years ago, long before the term "smoothie bowl" was coined, açaí bowls were the only game in town. I used to think "Is it just me, or is that just a thick smoothie served in a bowl?" So I started playing with smoothie bowls and came to love them. Don't get me wrong, I love a good açaí bowl too, but it's fun to mix things up! In this chapter I'm going to share a few of my favorite bowl recipes with some recommended topping options. I hope you love these recipes as much as I do.

<u>NOTE</u>: The same Dos and Don'ts from chapter 6 (smoothies) apply to bowls.

VANILLA DREAMS

Why you should eat this: Protein, antioxidants, magnesium, potassium, vitamin E, heart healthy and may improve digestion.

Reminiscent of a bowl of vanilla ice cream, but a whole lot healthier and, in my opinion, a whole lot tastier!

INGREDIENTS:

1 CUP
Frozen Banana

1 CUP
Ice

2 LARGE
Medjool Dates, pitted

3/4 CUPS
Sprouted Vanilla Almond Milk

1 TBSP
Almond Butter

1 TBSP
Choice Superfood Protein
(available in stores or online)

1/4 TSP
Cinnamon

TOPPING OPTIONS:

1/2 CUP
Choice Superseed Granola
(available in stores or online)

1/2
Fresh Banana, sliced

1 TBSP
Peanut Butter, drizzled
(or a scoop on top)

1 TBSP
Cacao Nibs
(for that extra cacao crunch)

PREPARATION:

01. Pre-blend the Sprouted Vanilla Almond Milk, dates, Choice Superfood Protein, cinnamon, and almond butter.

02. Add the frozen banana and ice and blend until an ice cream consistency is achieved. You may need to stop the blender and stir things around a bit, then continue blending until you reach a perfect, creamy texture. Remember, the less you blend, the thicker the smoothie bowl, and we want this smoothie bowl THICK! Don't over blend!

03. Pour into a bowl and add your favorite toppings! This smoothie bowl is delicious with granola, fresh slices of banana, peanut butter, and cacao nibs!

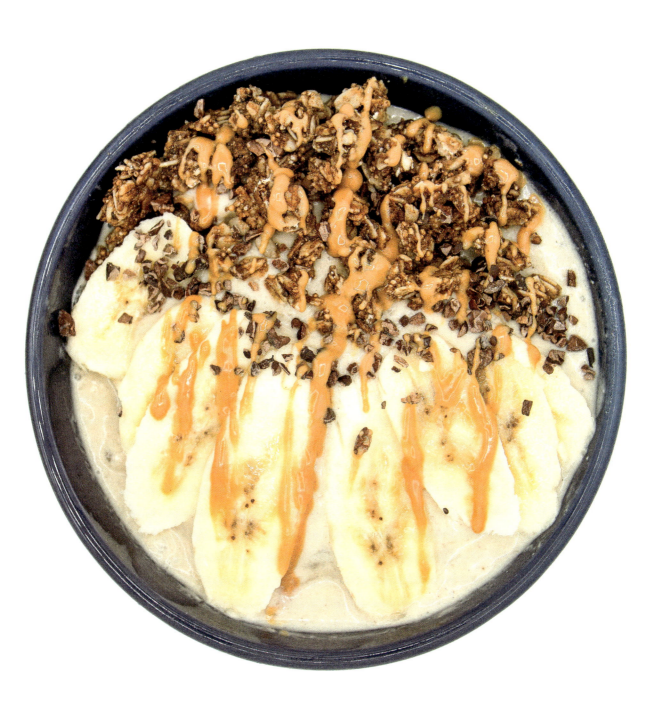

THE UNICORN

Why you should eat this: This smoothie bowl is rich with antioxidants, omega-3s, vitamins A and B12, and iron. It's packed with protein, may improve digestion, and is detoxifying, heart healthy, and has anti-inflammatory properties. Also, it's gorgeous!

I love food that tastes good, is aesthetically pleasing and is packed with nutrition. This Unicorn smoothie bowl is all of the above and then some! The beautiful blue and pink swirls give this bowl it's special name, "The Unicorn" which also happens to be available on the secret menu at Choice!

INGREDIENTS:

1 CUP
Frozen Banana

1 CUP
Frozen Strawberries

¾ CUP
Sprouted Vanilla Almond Milk

2 LARGE
Medjool Dates, pitted

1 TBSP
Choice Superfood Protein
(available online or in stores)

½ TSP
E3Live Blue Majik

TOPPING OPTIONS:

½ CUP
Choice Superseed Granola
(available in stores or online)

½
Fresh Banana, sliced

¼ CUP
Fresh Blueberries
        OR
¼ CUP
Strawberries, sliced

PREPARATION:

01. Pre-blend the Sprouted Vanilla Almond Milk, dates and Choice Superfood Protein.

02. Add the frozen bananas and strawberries and blend until a thick ice cream like consistency is achieved. You may need to stop the blender a couple of times and mix everything up a bit to get a smooth texture. Once the smoothie bowl is perfectly blended, add the E3Live Blue Majik and fold into the smoothie to create a majik swirl.

03. Carefully pour into a bowl and take it to the next level by adding granola, bananas, and fresh blueberries or strawberries!

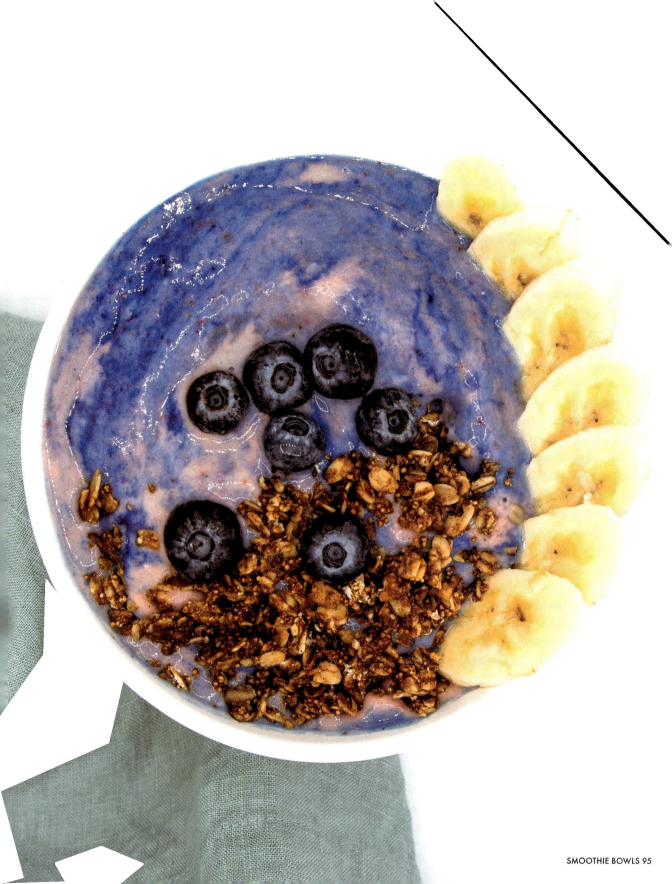

LEGEND

...smoothie bowl is alkalizing, high in protein, fiber, iron, and omega-3s. ...-boosting with a high mineral content, plus has fat-burning benefits, may ...inflammatory properties. This is the stuff legends are made of!

INGREDIENTS:

1 CUP
Frozen Banana

1 CUP
Ice

3/4 CUP
Sprouted Vanilla Almond Milk (or Oat Milk)

2 LARGE
Medjool Dates, pitted

1 TBSP
Choice Superfood Protein (available online or in stores)

1 TSP
Spirulina

1/2 CUP
Spinach (about a handful)

1 TBSP
Coconut Butter

1 TBSP
Hemp Seeds

PREPARATION:

01. Pre-blend the Sprouted Vanilla Almond Milk, dates, spirulina, Choice Superfood Protein, spinach, coconut butter and hemp seeds.

02. Add the frozen banana and ice and blend until an ice cream consistency is achieved. You may need to stop the blender and stir things around a bit, then continue blending until you reach a perfect, creamy texture. Remember, the less you blend, the thicker the smoothie bowl, and we want this smoothie bowl THICK! Don't over blend!

03. Pour into a bowl and add legendary toppings like granola, bananas, strawberries, and hemp seeds!

TOPPING OPTIONS:

1/2 CUP
Choice Superseed Granola (available in stores or online)

1/2
Fresh Banana, sliced

1/4 CUP
Strawberries, sliced

1 TBSP
Hemp Seeds

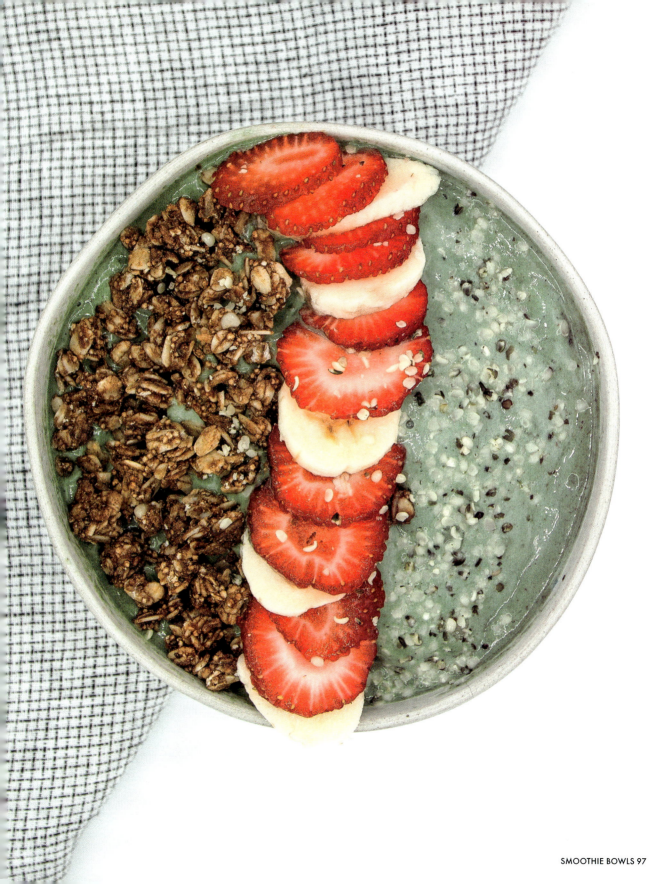

PEANUT BUTTER CRUNCH

Why you should eat this: Great for digestive health, high in protein, fiber, potassium, iron, calcium, great for heart health and may boost mood. It makes me happy just thinking about it!

INGREDIENTS:

1 CUP
Frozen Banana

1 CUP
Ice

3/4 CUP
Sprouted Vanilla Almond Milk
(or Oat Milk)

2 LARGE
Medjool Dates, pitted

1 TBSP
Choice Superfood Protein
(available online or in stores)

1 TBSP
Creamy Peanut Butter

1 TBSP
Cacao Nibs

TOPPING OPTIONS:

1/2 CUP
Choice Superseed Granola
(available in stores or online)

1/2
Fresh Banana, sliced

1/4 CUP
Strawberries, sliced

1 TBSP
Cacao Nibs
(for that extra cacao crunch)

PREPARATION:

01. Pre-blend the Sprouted Vanilla Almond Milk, dates, Choice Superfood Protein, and creamy peanut butter.

02. Toss in the frozen bananas and ice, and blend until an ice cream like consistency is achieved. You may need to stop the blender and stir things around a bit to get everything smooth. It's supposed to be thick, and it may take a minute, but trust me, it's worth it!

03. Add the Cacao Nibs and blend just until the nibs break into smaller pieces, about 4 seconds. If you like larger or smaller cacao nibs in your smoothie bowl, blend for a few seconds more or a few seconds less. Be careful though! The longer you blend, the thinner your smoothie bowl will become.

04. Add your toppings! Like the recipe mentions, I love this Peanut Butter Crunch topped with granola, fresh slices of strawberries and bananas, and extra nibs for that extra crunch!

THE COFFEE BEAN

Why you should eat this: Coffee and cinnamon are especially high in antioxidants and cinnamon is great for heart health. The Cold-Pressed Coffee and maca combo in this smoothie bowl are going to give you a nice burst of energy, and maca is awesome for hormone balancing, mood enhancing, and libido boosting! This may not be the best thing to enjoy before bed, but then again, maybe it is? Wink wink. ;)

INGREDIENTS:

1 CUP
Frozen Banana

1 CUP
Ice

3 OZ.
Sprouted Vanilla Almond Milk (or Oat Milk)

3 OZ.
Cold-Pressed Coffee

2 LARGE
Medjool Dates, pitted

1 TBSP
Choice Superfood Protein
(available in stores or online)

1 TSP
Maca Powder

1/8 TSP
Cinnamon

TOPPING OPTIONS:

1/2 CUP
Choice Superseed Granola
(available in stores or online)

1/2
Fresh Banana, sliced

1-2 TBSP
Peanut Butter, drizzled over the top

PREPARATION:

01. Pre-blend the Sprouted Vanilla Almond Milk, Cold-Pressed Coffee, dates, Choice Superfood Protein, cinnamon and maca.

02. Add the frozen banana and ice and blend until an ice cream consistency is achieved. You may need to stop the blender and stir things around a bit, then continue blending until you reach a perfect, creamy texture. Remember, the less you blend, the thicker the smoothie bowl, and we want this smoothie bowl THICK! Don't over blend!

03. Add whatever toppings you are craving! I love The Coffee Bean smoothie bowl topped with granola, fresh slices of banana, and a drizzle of creamy peanut butter! Yum!

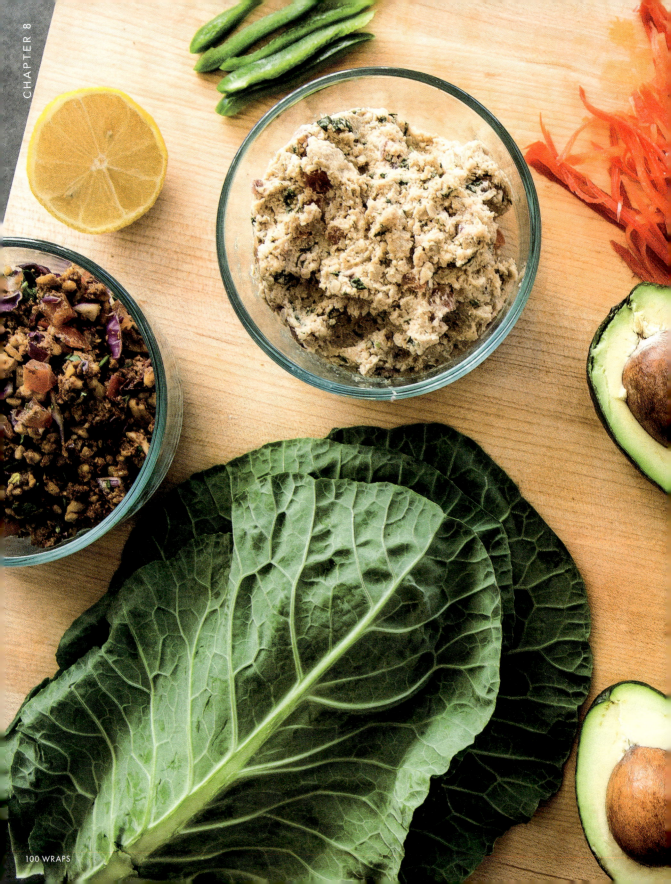

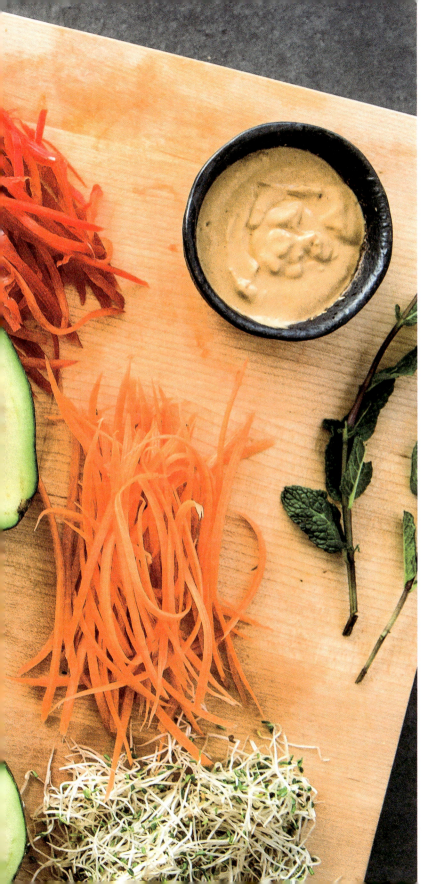

WRAPS

I love collard greens! So many nutrients and so few calories! Collards are an excellent source of vitamin A, vitamin C, vitamin K, and vitamin B-6. They contain lots of iron and magnesium, along with thiamin, niacin, pantothenic acid, and choline… I know, I had you at pantothenic acid. In other words, eat your greens–collard greens, that is!

WRAPS 101

PREPARATION FOR ALL WRAPS

Select large, fresh collard leaves. The bigger the collards, the easier to use for wraps! Wash and soak your collards in warm water with the juice of about ½ a lemon. This helps soften up the leaves and makes them pliable enough to roll. Place the washed collard greens on a cutting board and cut off the large stems at the base of the leaf. Then use a knife to thinly shave along the rib of the stem, starting at the base and moving up towards the top. After the collards are cleaned and soaked, and the stem and rib is removed, you are ready to roll!

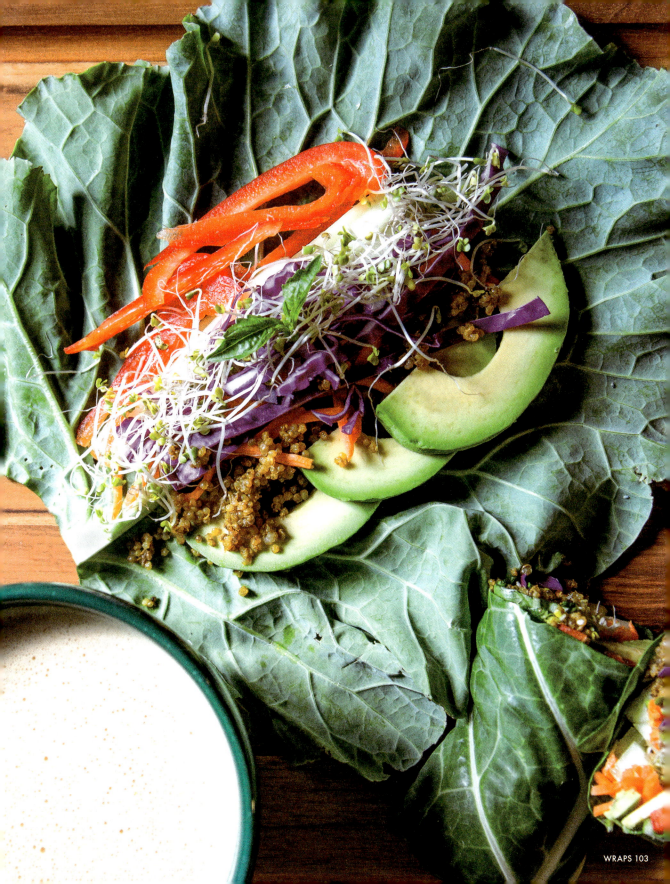

SPICY SUNTUNA WRAP with NACHO "CHEESE" DIPPING SAUCE

(MAKES 4 WRAPS)

This is my version of vegan tuna. Before going vegan, I used to love spicy tuna ceviche! This spicy suntuna pâté really hits the spot when that craving strikes!

WRAP INGREDIENTS:

2 CUPS
Spicy Suntuna Pâté
(SEE RECIPE TO THE RIGHT)

1 CUP
Nacho "Cheese" Sauce
(SERVED ON THE SIDE. SEE PG. 193)

4 LARGE
Collard Greens, prepared
(SEE PREPARATION ON PG. 102)

1 SMALL
Avocado, salted & cut into slices

1 CUP
Alfalfa Sprouts
(or Spring Mix)

½
Jalapeño, seeded and cut into thin matchsticks

¼ CUP
Purple Cabbage, shredded

SPICY SUNTUNA PÂTÉ (MAKES 2 CUPS)
INGREDIENTS:

1ST SET:

2 TBSP
Red Onion, diced

2 TBSP
Roma Tomatoes, diced

½
Jalapeño, seeded and diced

2 TBSP
Cilantro, chopped

2ND SET:

1 CUP
Sunflower Seeds, soaked in warm water for an hour

1 TBSP
Raw Cashews, soaked (you can combine the sunflower seeds and cashews when soaking)

2 TBSP
Olive Oil

2 TBSP
Lemon Juice

½ TSP
Himalayan Salt

½ TSP
Dulse Flakes (found at most health food stores)

½ TSP
Cayenne
(+ more if you desire a spicier "suntuna")

SPICY SUNTUNA PÂTÉ
PREPARATION:

01. Combine the first set of ingredients in a bowl.

02. Combine the soaked sunflower seeds and cashews with the oil, lemon juice and spices in a food processor and blend until a tuna salad-like consistency is achieved. The mixture should be light and fluffy, with few whole sunflower seeds remaining.

03. Once desired texture is achieved, empty the pâté into the bowl with the fresh vegetables and combine by hand.

WRAP
PREPARATION:

01. Prepare Spicy Suntuna Pâté and Nacho "Cheese" Sauce (see recipe on pg. 193)

02. Divide the Spicy Suntuna Pâté, avocado, alfalfa sprouts, cabbage, and sliced jalapeño between your four prepared collards. Roll one end of the collard leaf over the fillings lengthwise. Then fold the ends in, roll again, and place wrap seam-side down on a cutting board.

03. Slice in half and serve with Nacho "Cheese" Sauce, and enjoy.

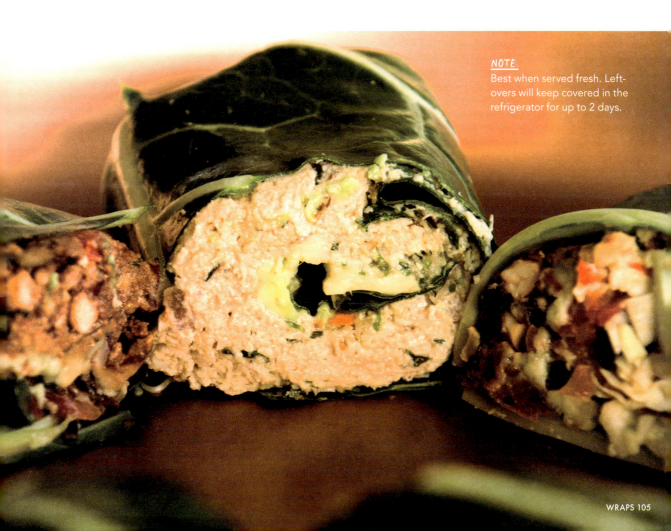

NOTE: Best when served fresh. Leftovers will keep covered in the refrigerator for up to 2 days.

WALNUT TACO "MEAT"

INGREDIENTS:

3 1/3 CUPS
Walnuts, finely chopped, or pulsed in a food processor

3/4 CUP
Sun Dried Tomatoes, or ½ cup tomato paste

2 TBSP
Gluten-Free Tamari

2 TSP
Water

1 TBSP
Cumin

1 TBSP
Onion Powder

1 TBSP
Paprika

1 TSP
Garlic Powder

2 TBSP
Nutritional Yeast

3/4 CUP
Cilantro

1/8 TSP
Himalayan Salt

PREPARATION:

01. Combine water, sun dried tomatoes or tomato paste, and tamari in a blender and blend until a smooth, thick paste is formed. Add more water as needed.

02. Remove paste from the blender, and place in a medium-sized bowl.

03. Add spices to the tomato/tamari paste and work with your hands until well incorporated.

04. Add walnuts and cilantro and mix well until combined.

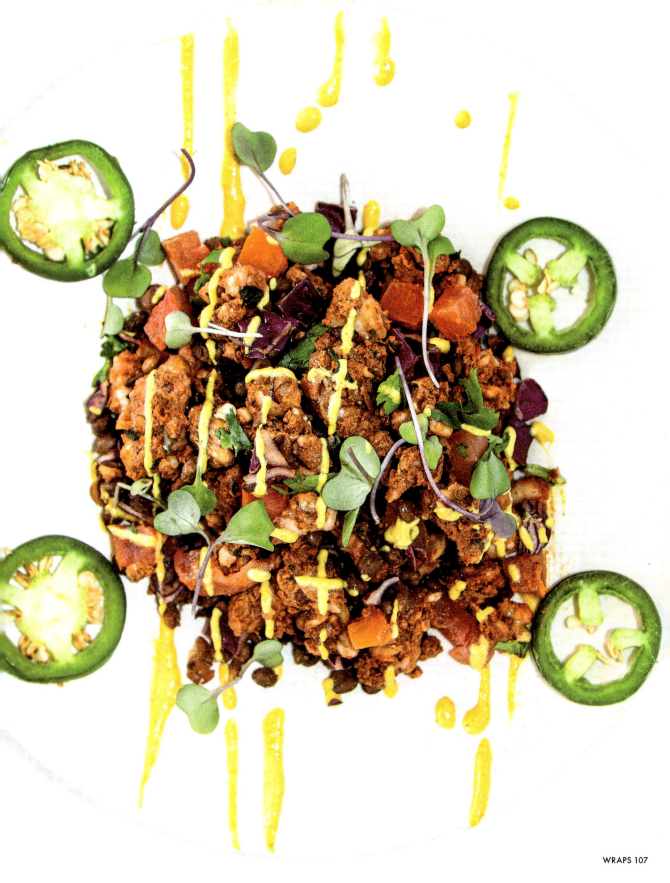

MACHO TACO COLLARD WRAP with CHIPOTLE "CHEESE" SAUCE (MAKES 4 WRAPS)

INGREDIENTS:

2 CUPS
Walnut Taco "Meat"
(SEE RECIPE ON PREVIOUS PAGE)

1 CUP
Chipotle "Cheese" Sauce
(served on the side, see recipe on pg. 192)

4 LARGE
Collard Greens, prepared
(SEE PREPARATION ON PG. 102)

1 CUP
Alfalfa, Broccoli,
or Radish Sprouts

½ CUP
Fresh Cilantro

1 RIPE
Avocado, sliced and salted

½ CUP
Red Onion, thinly sliced

PREPARATION:

01. Prepare Walnut Taco "Meat" and Chipotle "Cheese" Sauce, if you haven't already.

02. Place ½ cup of Walnut Taco "Meat" in each prepared collard wrap, and top with avocado, sliced onions, cilantro and sprouts. Roll one end of the collard leaf over the fillings lengthwise. Then fold the ends in, roll again, and place the wrap seam-side down.

03. Slice the collard wrap in half, and serve with Chipotle "Cheese" Sauce.

NOTE:
Best when served fresh. Leftovers will keep covered in the refrigerator for up to 2 days.

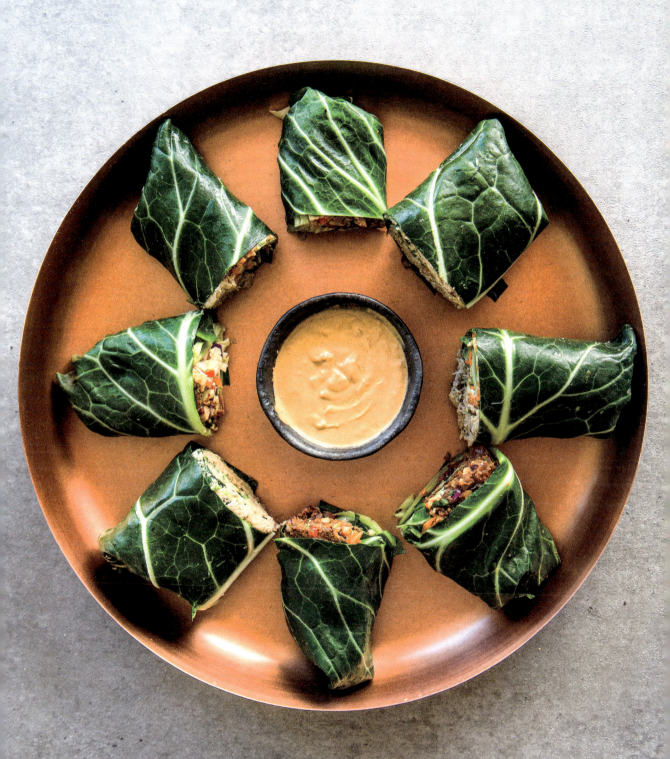

COLLARD SPRING ROLL with PAD THAI DIPPING SAUCE

INGREDIENTS:

4 LARGE
Collard Greens, prepared
(SEE PREPARATION ON PG. 102)

1 SMALL
Red Bell Pepper, cut into thin strips

1 SMALL
English Cucumber, cut into thin strips

1 SMALL
Carrot, cut into matchsticks

1 RIPE
Avocado, sliced and salted

1 CUP
Alfalfa Sprouts

½ CUP
Purple Cabbage, shredded

HANDFUL OF
Fresh Basil Leaves

1 CUP
Turmeric Quinoa
(SEE PREPARATION OF THE RIGHT)

1 CUP
Pad Thai Sauce
(FOR DIPPING. SERVED ON THE SIDE. SEE RECIPE ON PG. 205)

TURMERIC QUINOA
PREPARATION:

01. Add 1 tsp turmeric, 1 tsp salt, and 1 Tbsp olive oil to 1 cup of quinoa and prepare according to package directions. Set aside.

WRAP
PREPARATION:

01. Divide all ingredients evenly between your prepared collards. There's no exact measurement, so load 'em up to your heart's content!

02. Roll one end of the collard leaf over the fillings lengthwise. Then fold the ends in, roll again, and place wrap seam-side down on a cutting board.

03. Slice rolls in half and serve with Pad Thai sauce.

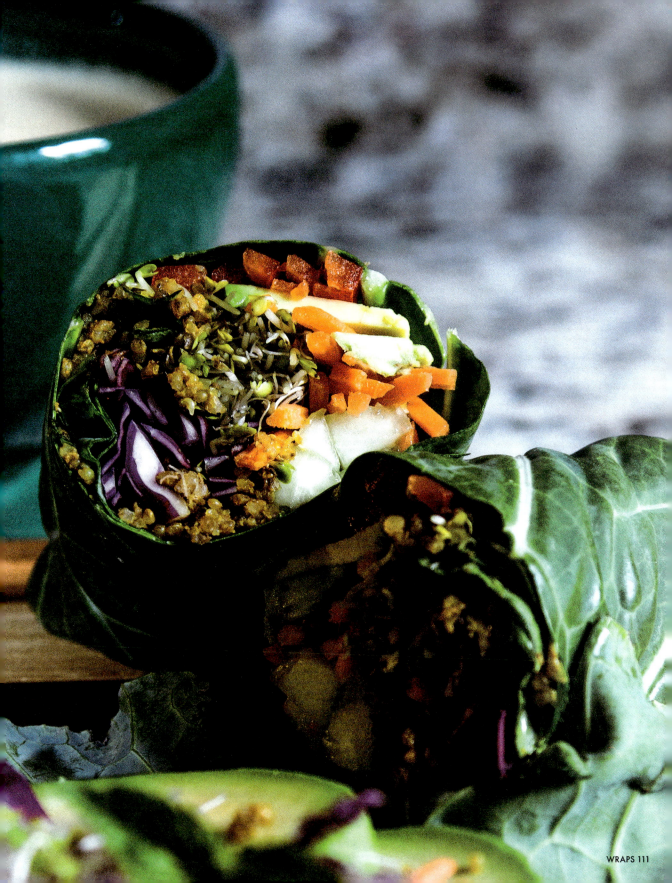

BBQ JACKFRUIT LETTUCE WRAP with VEGAN SLAW

BBQ JACKFRUIT
INGREDIENTS:

2 14 OZ. CANS
Green Jackfruit in brine
(rinsed and drained)

1 ½ CUPS
Choice BBQ Sauce
(SEE RECIPE ON PG. 200)

1 TBSP
Olive Oil

3 TBSP
Water

LETTUCE WRAPS
INGREDIENTS:

1 HEAD
Butter Lettuce

2 RIPE
Avocados, diced and salted

2 CUPS
Vegan Slaw
(SEE RECIPE ON PG. 208)

BBQ JACKFRUIT
PREPARATION:

01. In a sauté pan, heat olive oil over medium heat.

02. Add jackfruit and sauté for five minutes.

03. Add Choice BBQ sauce and water to the pan and stir to evenly coat jackfruit.

04. Cover pan and simmer on medium-low heat for 20-25 minutes, stirring occasionally and pulling jackfruit apart as it becomes tender.

LETTUCE WRAPS
PREPARATION:

01. Gently remove lettuce leaves, taking care not to tear them.

02. Rinse and pat dry butter lettuce leaves

03. Place a scoop of pulled BBQ jackfruit on top of your lettuce wrap.

04. Top with vegan slaw and diced avocado. Eat and repeat until satisfied!

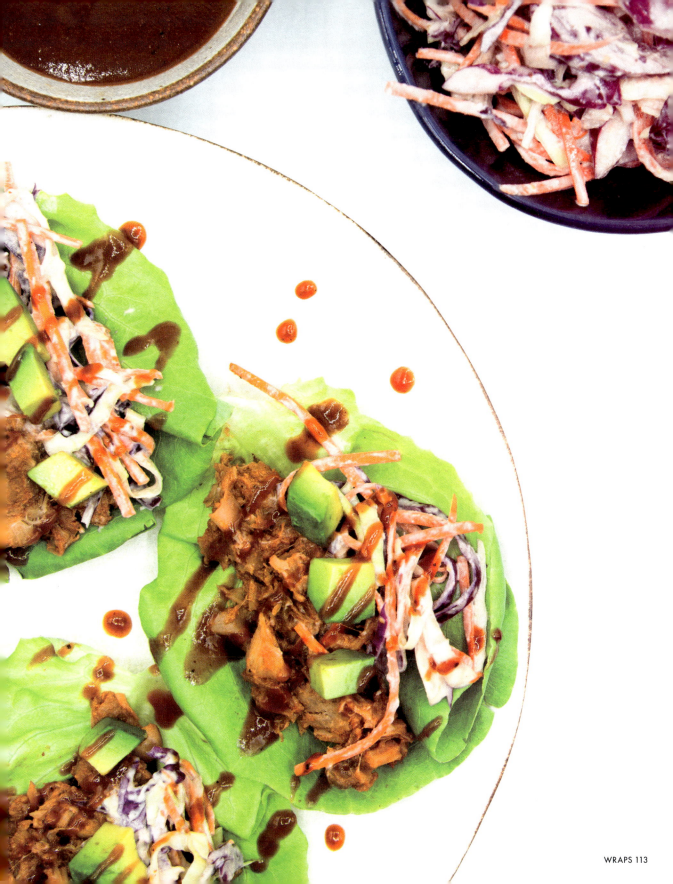

"CARNITAS" LETTUCE WRAPS

These "Carnitas" Wraps are so delicious. You can use your "carnitas" for tacos, burritos, bowls and so much more. Oyster mushrooms are a rich source of protein, vitamins, minerals, fiber, and antioxidants. They can protect the body's cells from damage that could lead to chronic diseases and are known to help strengthen the immune system. Oyster mushrooms are low in calories, they are fat free, cholesterol free, gluten-free, very low in sodium, and they are delicious! Truly perfect for this recipe, and should not be substituted for any other mushroom when making these "carnitas".

MUSHROOM "CARNITAS"
INGREDIENTS:

1 LB
Oyster Mushrooms, shredded

3 TBSP
Olive Oil

1 1/2 TSP
Chopped Garlic

1/2 TSP
Garlic Powder

3/4 TSP
Himalayan Salt

LETTUCE WRAPS

8 LEAVES
Butter Lettuce, rinsed and dried

1 RIPE
Avocado, sliced and salted

1/4 CUP
Chipotle "Cheese" Sauce
(SEE RECIPE ON PAGE 192)

1/4 CUP
Green Onion, sliced

1/2 CUP
Purple Cabbage, shredded

1/4 CUP
Cilantro, chopped

ADOBO SAUCE
INGREDIENTS:

2
Guajillo Chiles, soaked and drained

1 LARGE
Roma Tomato, diced

1/2 SMALL
Red Bell Pepper, chopped

2 TBSP
Yellow Onion, chopped

1 LARGE
Garlic Clove

1/8 TSP
Ground Clove

3
Black Pepper Corns

1/4 TSP
Fresh Oregano, chopped

1
Bay Leaf

1/2 TSP
Himalayan Salt

2 TSP
Maple Syrup

1/4 TSP
Cumin

1 TBSP
Lemon Juice

1 TSP
Apple Cider Vinegar

1/4 TSP
Onion Powder

TURN PAGE
FOR PREPARATION AND METHODS

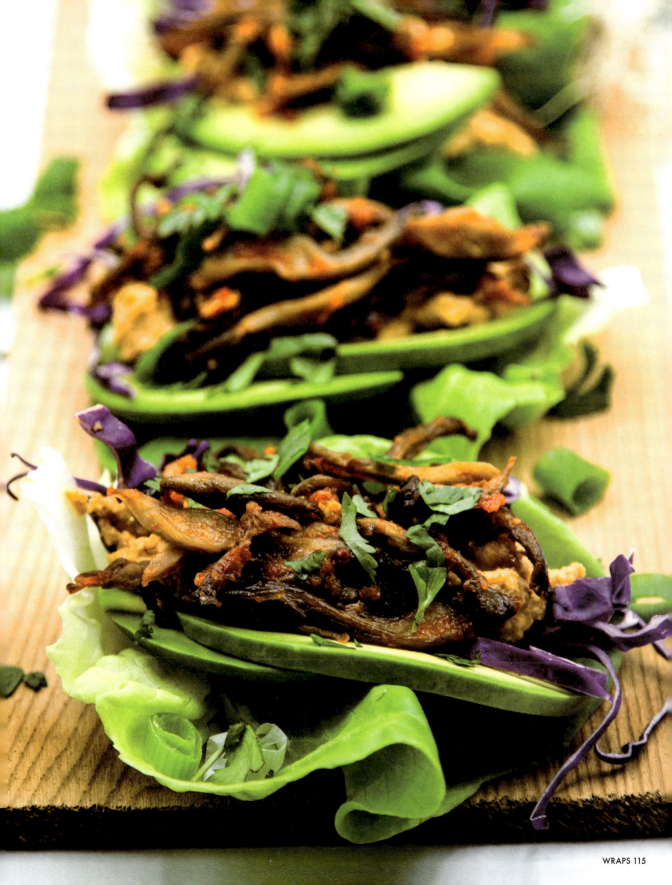

"CARNITAS"
PREPARATION:

01. Preheat the oven to 375° F.

02. Massage the shredded mushrooms with olive oil, chopped garlic, garlic powder and salt. Place on a baking sheet and cook for 12-18 mins (or until they begin to get a little charred and crispy).

03. Pour prepared adobo sauce over mushrooms and let marinade for 1 hour.

NOTE:
You may not need to use all of the adobo sauce. The goal is to fully cover the mushrooms, without drowning them. That being said, use your discretion as you add the sauce. I like having a little extra to drizzle on top of my lettuce wraps so I usually save a portion of the adobo sauce.

ADOBO SAUCE
PREPARATION:

01. Blend all adobo sauce ingredients in a high powered blender for 3-5 mins until completely puréed. Taste and adjust seasonings as needed. This will keep for up to a week in the fridge. It's great on top of the lettuce wraps, enchiladas, burrito bowls and more!

LETTUCE WRAPS

01. Portion your "carnitas" onto your lettuce wraps. Top with shredded cabbage, green onion, cilantro, and ripe avocado, and drizzle the Chipotle "cheese" sauce on top. Serve immediately.

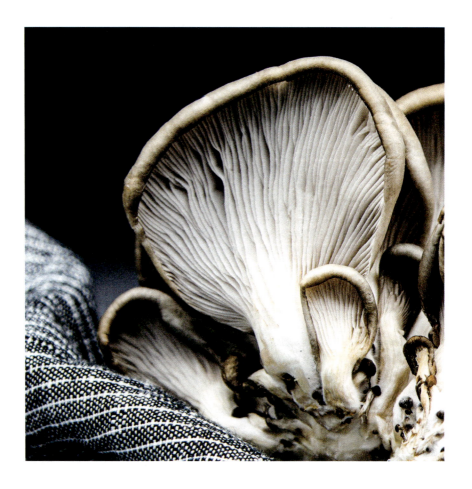

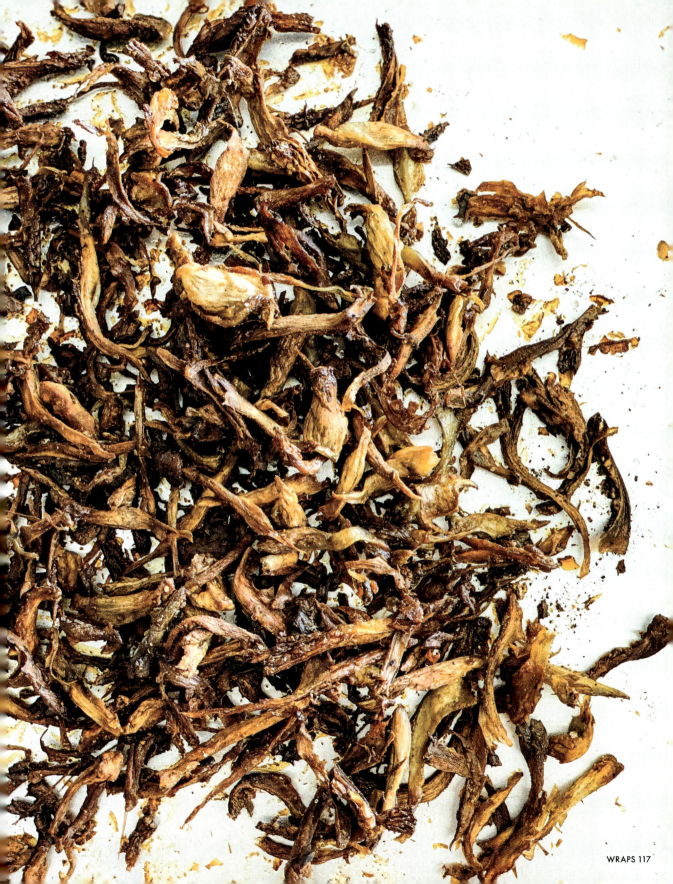

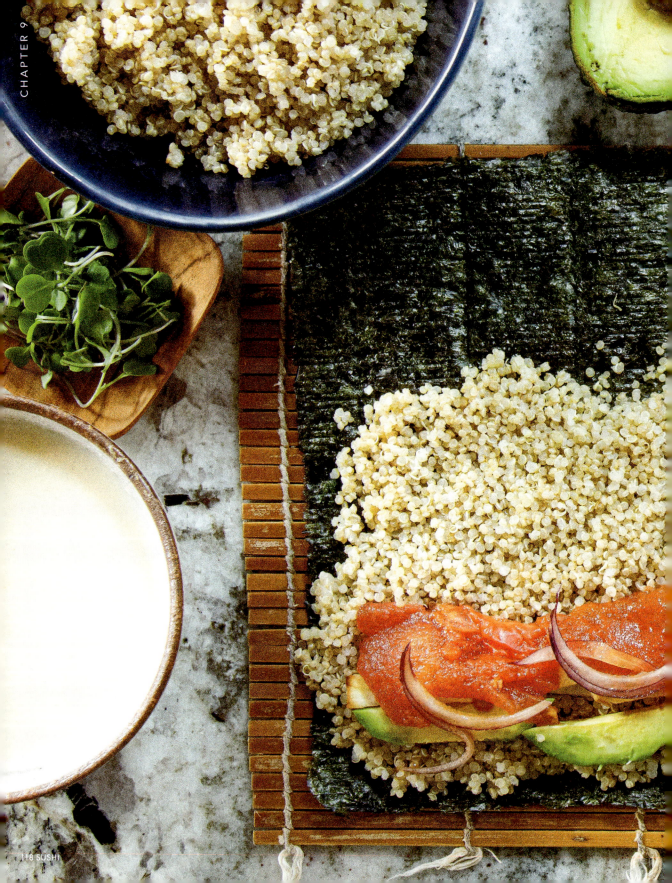

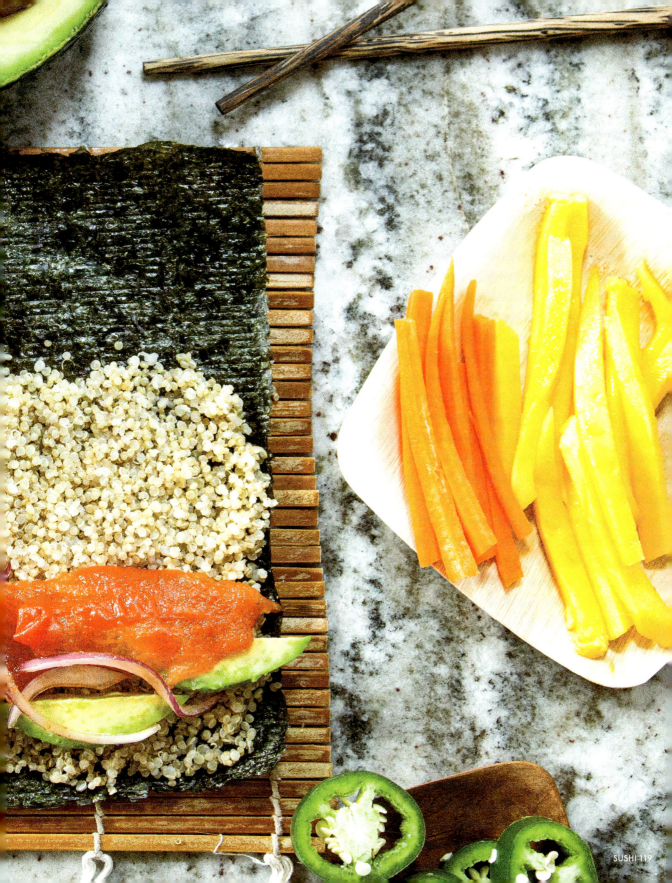

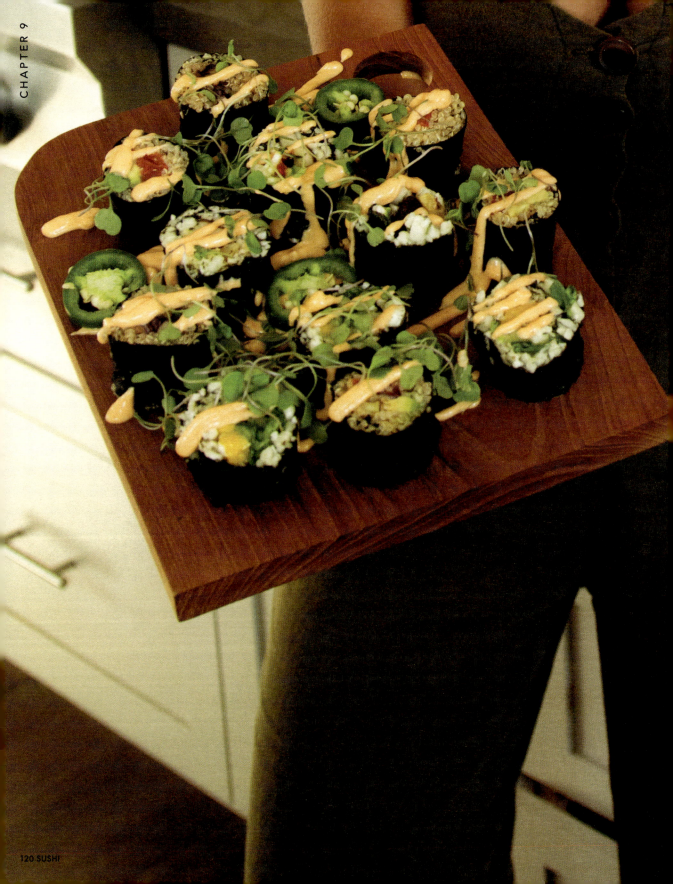

SUSHI

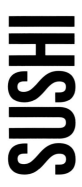

Sushi is such a fun food both to make, and to eat! People always think that I'm crazy when I say sushi is one of my favorite foods, considering I'm 100% plant-based! When most people think of sushi, they think it's exclusively composed of fish, but that's not actually the case. I'm excited to share some of my favorite plant-based (and healthy) rice-free versions of sushi with you! Note: you can absolutely sub rice into any of these recipes and they would be equally delicious. I just happen to love them as is.

Let's talk about methodology, because <u>this is going to be the foundation of all your rolls,</u> no matter what goodness you fill them with.

WHAT YOU NEED:

01. Sushi Mat— You can find sushi mats at any Asian food market, some health food markets and you can also order them online as well.

02. A Good Sharp Knife— A carving knife will work, and a serrated knife can work as well if you cut slowly in a sawing motion.

PREPARATION:

01. First, you'll want to wrap your sushi mat in plastic wrap, completely covering the bamboo mat so that no "rice" or nori touch the mat. Then place a sheet of nori flat onto your sushi mat, rough side facing UP.

02. Add some cauliflower rice (or quinoa, depending on the recipe you are using) on the bottom half of the nori and top with remaining ingredients for your specific roll (specific measurements of each ingredient are included in the recipe section of this chapter). Each ingredient should be in its own line, on top of the "cauliflower rice."

<u>NOTE</u>:
The goal here is consistency. You're going to be chopping this sushi roll into bite-size pieces and you want each piece to have very similar ingredients. Keep that in mind as you're placing the remaining ingredients on top of the "rice."

03. Beginning on the side with the filling (bottom half), use the mat to begin rolling the nori up over the filling. Use your fingers to guide it and help "smush" the ingredients together in the roll.

04. Continue to roll the sushi. Tuck the front edge of the nori into the roll, and remove the mat as you continue to roll the sushi. Roll slowly so that you ensure that the sushi is coming out even.

05. Tighten the roll to keep ingredients from falling out when you cut it. Remember to tighten the roll with your sushi mat often, but not too tightly. Roll the sushi roll back and forth in the mat to tighten and seal it.

06. Cut the roll into sixths or eighths using a sharp, wet knife. The thickness of the slices is determined by the number of ingredients. If you have more ingredients in the roll, the slices should be thinner for ease in enjoying.

07. Serve your sushi immediately. Sushi is best when eaten freshly-made.

Now that you know HOW it's done, it's time for the mouth-watering recipes!

SPICY "AHI"

"THIS IS ONE OF MY BEST KEPT SECRETS."

I love making "poke" bowls and spicy "tuna" rolls for family dinners and gatherings because of the star of both of these dishes, which is always a hit.

People always ask me what I use to make "tuna" and it's way simpler than you think! I hate to sell it short by saying "it's just tomato" but the truth is, it's just tomato! The magic comes from the preparation. The tomatoes need to be boiled, peeled, filleted and marinated for hours prior. This process is what gives the tomatoes a resemblance in taste and texture to it's fishy counterpart (minus the fishy taste).

INGREDIENTS:

- 6 LARGE Tomatoes
- 1/4 CUP Gluten-Free Tamari
- 1/4 CUP Ponzu (organic and vegan)
- 1 TBSP Rice Vinegar
- 1/4 CUP Green Onion
- 1/4 CUP Red Onion (very thinly sliced)
- 1 TSP Pure Maple Syrup
- 1 TBSP Lemon Juice
- 1 TSP Onion Powder
- 1 TSP Garlic Powder
- 2 TSP Sesame Oil
- 2 TBSP Olive Oil
- 1 TBSP Chili Sauce (if you like it spicy)
- 1 TBSP Ginger, freshly grated
- 1 TBSP Nutritional Yeast

PREPARATION:

01. Mix all ingredients (except tomatoes) into a large bowl and set aside.

02. Add your tomatoes to a pot of boiling water. When the tomato skins start to crack open, turn the water off. Let it sit for another minute or two, but no more than that or you will have mush!

03. Strain the tomatoes and rinse them with cold water for a few minutes so you can work with them without burning your hands. Carefully peel away the skin. It should come right off.

04. Next, cut them in half, then in half again (quartering each tomato). Take your knife and run it along the inside of each quarter, removing the seeds and reserving the flesh, leaving a nice clean filet. As you do this, place each individual filet into your marinade.

05. Once you've finished all of your tomatoes, cover your bowl and place in the fridge for a minimum of 20 minutes (up to overnight). The longer the Spicy "Ahi" sits in the marinade, the better the sushi.

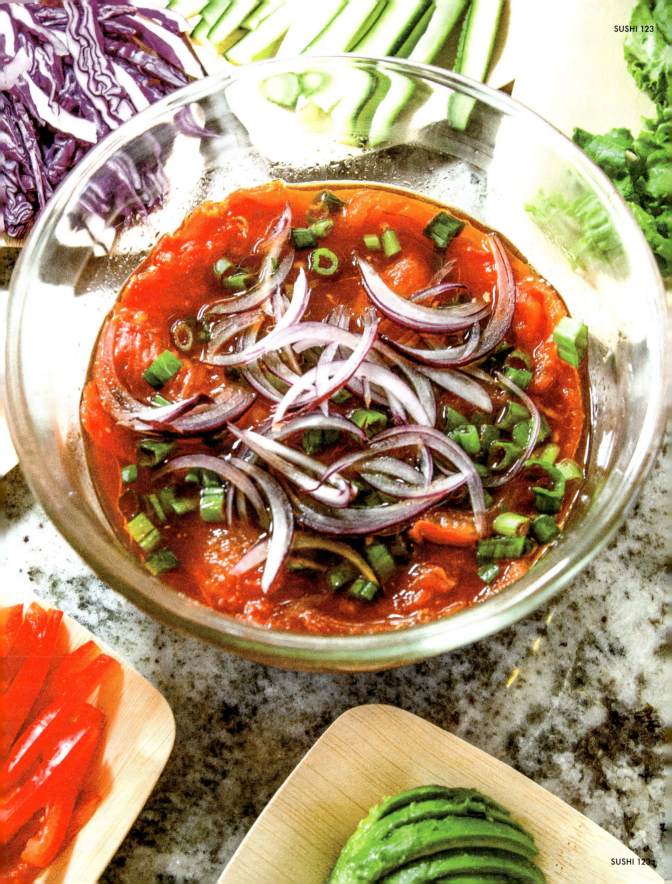

PORTOBELLO QUINOA SUSHI ROLL

This is such a great roll! Maki style—making it super easy to prep. I love finding ways to get mushrooms in my diet because they are such an excellent source of nutrition (and they are equally delicious).

Portobello mushrooms, like so many other mushrooms, have a rich array of vitamins and nutrients that boost your immune system, including potentially fighting and preventing certain cancers. They are rich in some of the B vitamins – riboflavin, niacin (vitamin B3), and pantothenic acid. Portobello mushrooms offer high antioxidant and anti-inflammatory properties while remaining low fat, low carb, and low calorie. They're also an excellent source of selenium, a critical mineral that helps the human body produce thyroid hormones, supports the immune system, and offers protection against heart disease.

INGREDIENTS:
MAKES 2 ROLLS

2 SHEETS
Nori

2 CUPS
Sushi Quinoa
(SEE RECIPE TO THE RIGHT)

5 OZ.
Portobello Mushrooms, marinated (SEE RECIPE TO THE RIGHT)

½ LARGE
Avocado, sliced and salted

4 OZ.
Miso Ginger Dressing
(SEE RECIPE ON PG. 204)

1
Jalapeño, sliced to serve on top or on the side (deseed to remove heat)

OPTIONAL:
Wasabi sprouts for garnish or other micro green of choice

SUSHI QUINOA
INGREDIENTS:

1 CUP
Uncooked Quinoa, rinsed well

1 ½ CUPS
Water

½ CUP
Rice Vinegar

2 TSP
Agave or Pure Maple Syrup

2 TSP
Himalayan Salt

SUSHI QUINOA
PREPARATION:

01. Add the quinoa and water to a medium saucepan set over high heat. Bring to a boil, then lower the heat and cover. Simmer until the quinoa is mostly cooked through but still on the undercooked side, about 15-20 minutes. The water will have absorbed but the quinoa won't quite be translucent.

02. Meanwhile, set a small saucepan over medium heat and add the rice vinegar, maple syrup (or agave) and Himalayan salt. Bring just to a simmer and keep warm until the quinoa is ready.

03. Pour the vinegar mixture into the pan with the quinoa, stir well, cover and let sit until the quinoa absorbs the liquid.

04. Remove the quinoa from the heat and let it cool completely. I like to add the vinegar mixture a little at a time, tasting as I go. I suggest doing this so you get the desired flavor.

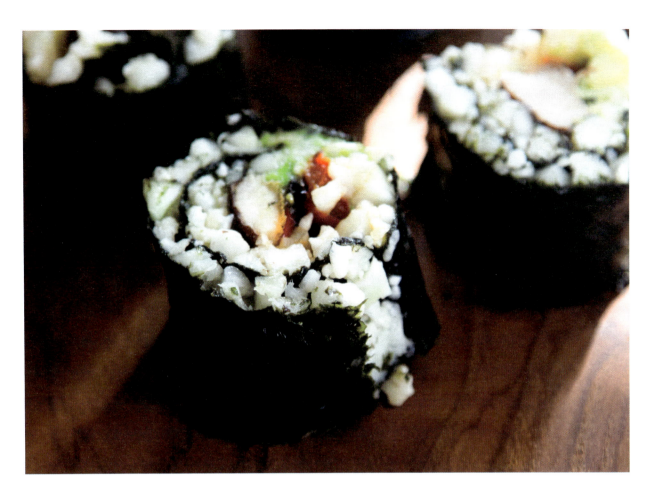

MUSHROOM MARINADE
INGREDIENTS:

(PREP A DAY IN ADVANCE FOR BEST RESULTS)

1 ½ LBS
Portobello Mushrooms, stems removed and sliced
(about 4-5 large Portobello caps)

½ CUP
Gluten-Free Tamari

¼ CUP
Sesame Oil

¾ TSP
Onion Powder

¼ TSP
Garlic Powder

MUSHROOM MARINADE
PREPARATION:

01. Combine all ingredients in a large bowl.

02. Cover and refrigerate for at least an hour before using, but for best results, prep a day in advance.

*follow the prep instructions for rolling found in the beginning of this chapter.

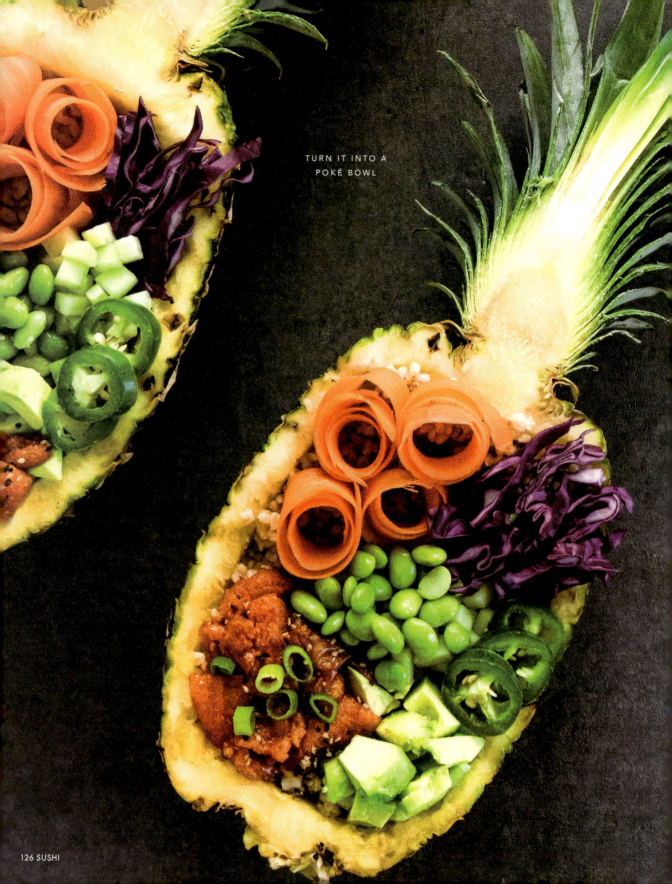

TURN IT INTO A
POKÉ BOWL

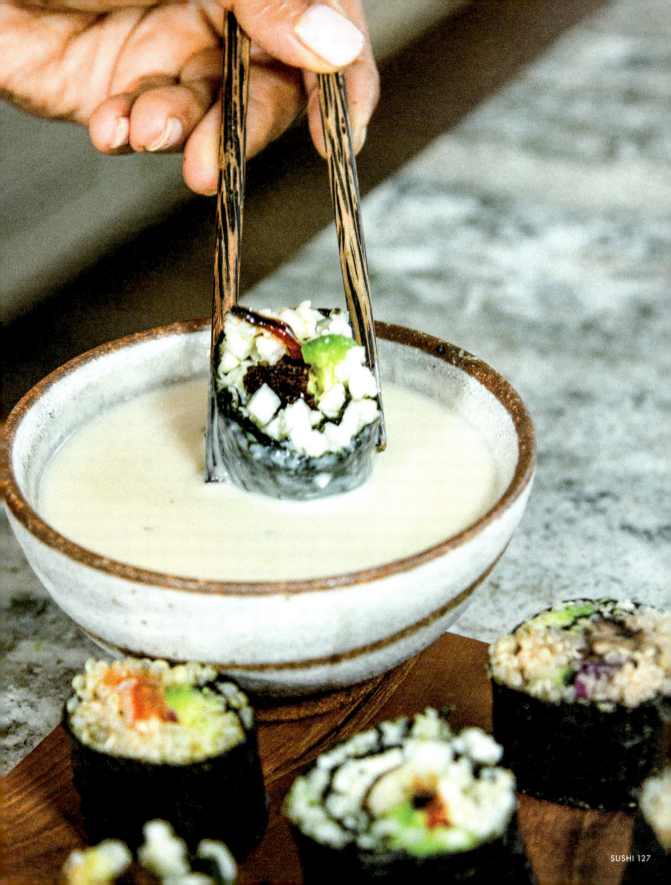

SPICY AVOCADO MANGO ROLL

This roll is also delicious with the Spicy Cashew Aioli or the Miso Ginger Dipping Sauce (both recipes in chapter 15) either served on the side, or drizzled on top. It's always fun to toss your microgreens on top of all of your rolls for a great presentation and a ton of nutrition.

INGREDIENTS:
(MAKES 1 ROLL)

1 SHEET
Nori

3 SLICES
Mango

3 SLICES
Cucumber

3 SLICES
Avocado, salted

3 SLICES
Jalapeño, julienned
(OPTIONAL IF YOU LIKE IT SPICY)

¾ CUP
Cauliflower Sushi Rice
(SEE RECIPE ON PG. 132)

Microgreens
(OPTIONAL GARNISH)

PREPARATION:

*follow the prep instructions for rolling found in the beginning of this chapter.

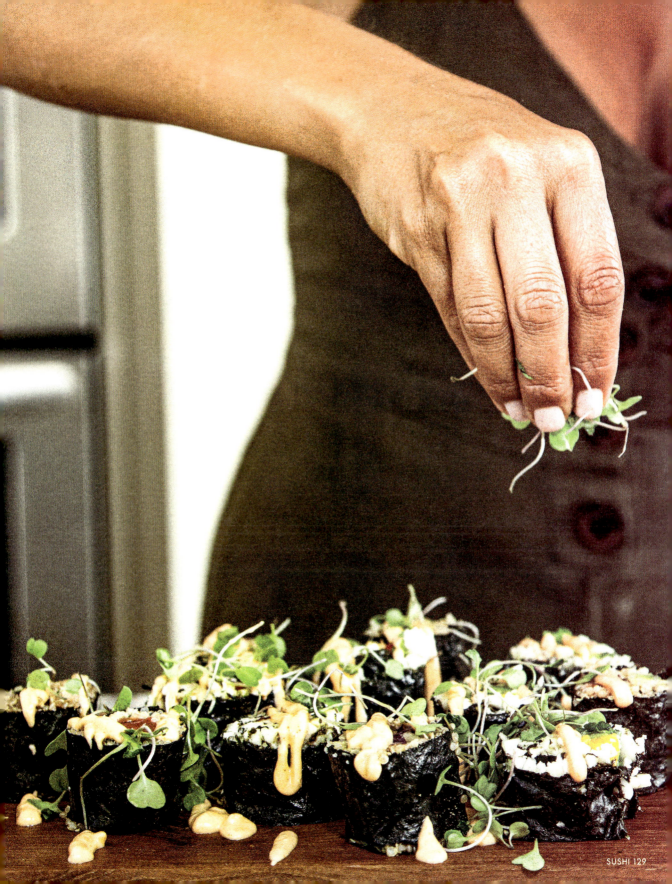

"AHI" ROLL with SPICY CASHEW AIOLI (MAKI STYLE)

This is one of my favorite rolls to make for friends. They are always blown away by the texture and flavor of the "ahi." It has to be made maki style with the sushi quinoa, unless you swap out for traditional sushi rice.

INGREDIENTS:
(MAKES 1 ROLL)

1 SHEET
Nori

1 CUP
Sushi Quinoa
(SEE RECIPE ON PG. 124)

3
Spicy "Ahi" Fillets, squeeze to drain sauce before placing in roll.
(SEE SPICY "AHI" RECIPE PG. 122)

3 SLICES
Avocado, salted

3 SLICES
Sweet Potato, roasted
(SEE PREPARATION TO THE RIGHT)

Spicy Cashew Aioli
(SEE RECIPE ON PG. 205)

"AHI" ROLL
PREPARATION:

01. Using a piping tool (or a ziplock with the corner snipped off), fill the bag with Spicy Cashew Aioli.

02. Roll sushi, slice, and drizzle the Spicy Cashew Aioli all over your freshly prepared roll and serve immediately.

*follow the prep instructions for rolling found in the beginning of this chapter.

ROASTED SWEET POTATO
PREPARATION:

01. 1 Sweet potato cut lengthwise into fries, tossed in olive oil, salt and garlic.

02. Roast for 30-40 minutes at 400°F degrees (this will make enough for 5-8 rolls depending on size)

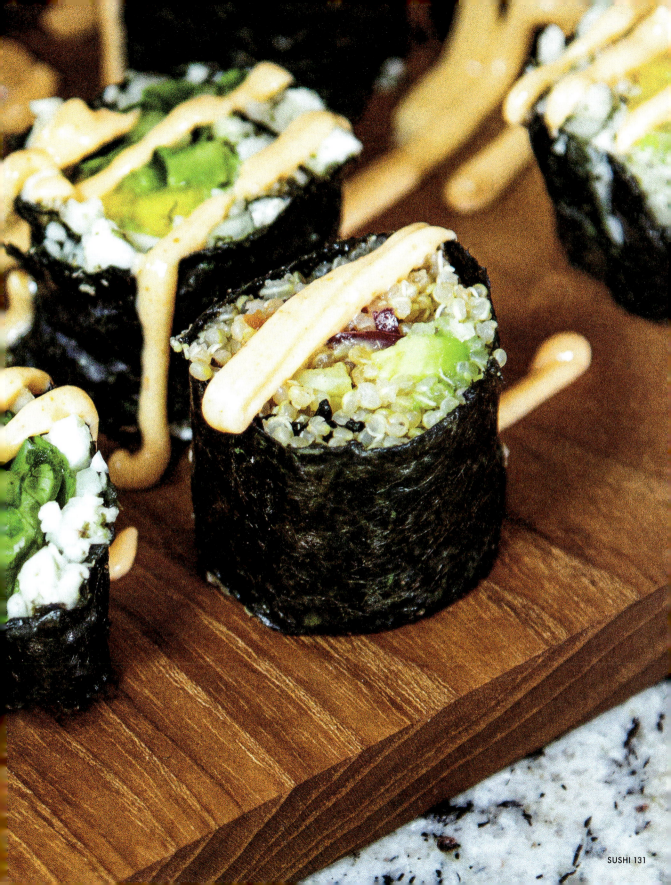

CAULIFLOWER SUSHI RICE

Cauliflower is loaded with nutrients, is anti-inflammatory, has anti-aging properties and can aid in weight loss, among many other benefits.

Using cauliflower in place of rice when making sushi is a brilliant way to get more veggies into your diet- and enjoy sushi at the same time!

One large head of cauliflower will give you roughly 3 cups of "rice," depending on the size of the cauliflower. This should be enough for a few rolls. Cauliflower isn't sticky or wet, which is what makes rolling sushi with it a bit tricky. For this reason, we are going to dress this cauliflower rice, which will also add a nice little boost of flavor to your rolls.

INGREDIENTS:

1 LARGE
Cauliflower (or 2 small heads of cauliflower)

2 TBSP
Rice Vinegar

1 TBSP
Miso (I like chickpea miso)

1 TBSP
Lemon Juice

1/8 TSP
Himalayan Salt (more to taste)

1 TSP
Agave

DIRECTIONS:

01. There are two techniques for making cauliflower rice. You can either use a box grater with the medium-size holes, traditionally used for cheese. Or a food processor with the grater blade to blitz it into small pieces. With both techniques, you're aiming for little pieces the size of rice.

02. Once you've got your "rice" ready, place it into a bowl and add all ingredients above. Then, using your hands, massage through the rice giving it a squeeze every now and again to make sure it's really picking up the moisture thoroughly.

03. Now you're ready to roll - your sushi that is!

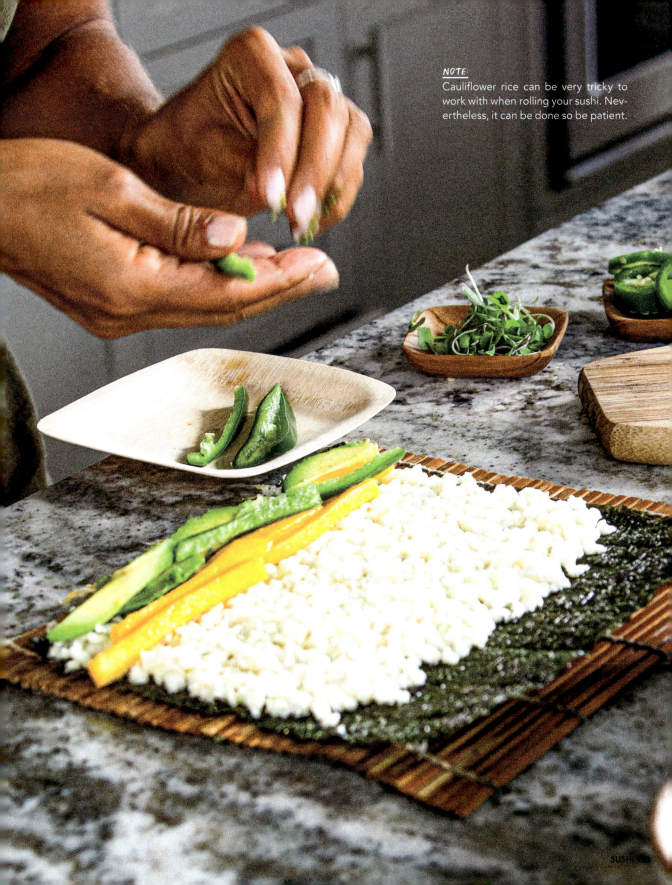

NOTE:
Cauliflower rice can be very tricky to work with when rolling your sushi. Nevertheless, it can be done so be patient.

SHIITAKE ROLL

I typically make several different rolls when I make sushi. That being said, the quantity below is for an individual roll, but you can roast a lot more of the individual ingredients as you will use these in several different rolls.

INGREDIENTS:

½ CUP
Shiitake Mushrooms, roasted
(SEE RECIPE TO THE RIGHT)

2-3 SLICES
Sweet Potato, roasted

3 SLICES
Avocado, salted

3 SLICES
Red Bell Pepper, roasted and julienned

1 CUP
Sushi Quinoa (SEE RECIPE ON PG. 124 - OR USE THE RECIPE FOR CAULIFLOWER SUSHI RICE ON PG. 132)

OPTIONAL:
Drizzle with Miso Ginger Sauce or Spicy Cashew Aioli

PREPARATION:

FOR THE SWEET POTATO:

01. Cut 1 sweet potato into long strips, like sweet potato fries. Toss in olive oil and salt.

02. Roast for 30-40 minutes at 400°F degrees (this will make enough for 5-8 rolls depending on size)

FOR THE MUSHROOMS:

01. 1 cup Shiitake mushrooms (stems removed) cut into strips. Toss in olive oil, salt and garlic powder.

02. Roast for 20-30 mins at 375°F (this is enough for about 2-3 rolls).

FOR THE BELL PEPPER:

01. 1 Red bell pepper cut into long strips. Toss in olive oil and salt.

02. Roast in the oven for 30 mins at 375°F (this is enough for 4 + rolls).

 *follow the prep instructions for rolling found in the beginning of this chapter.

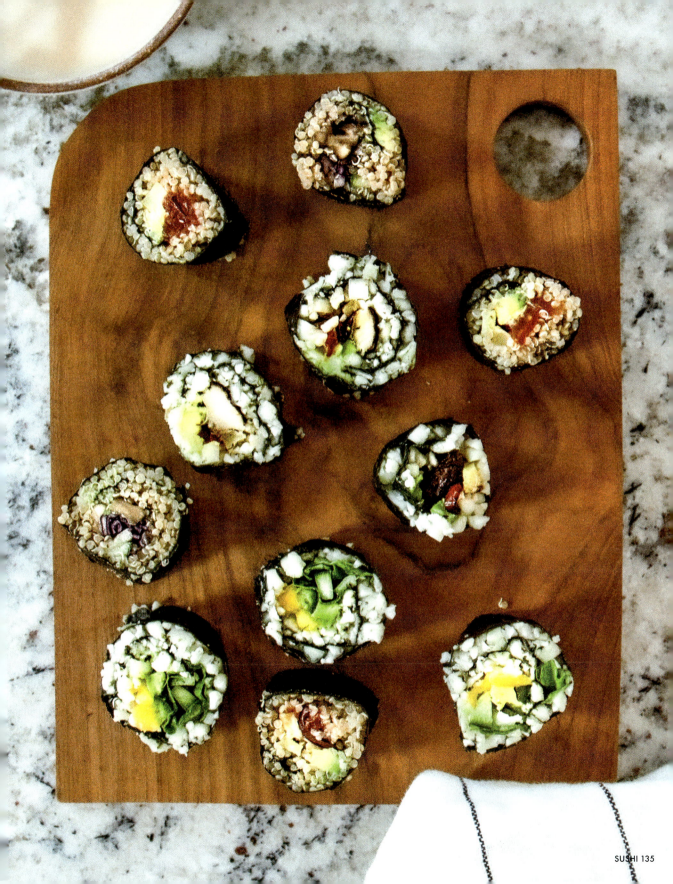

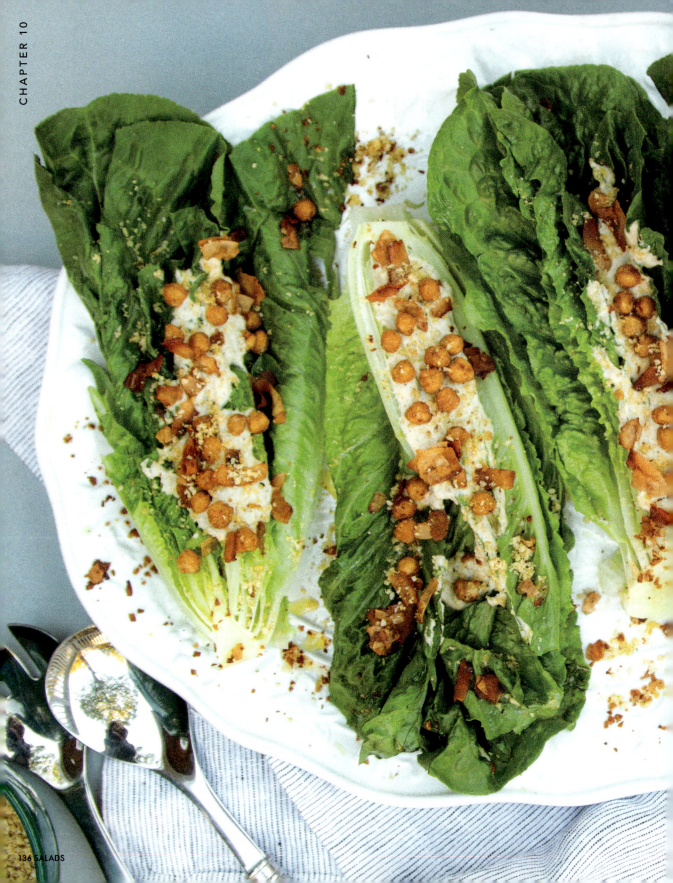

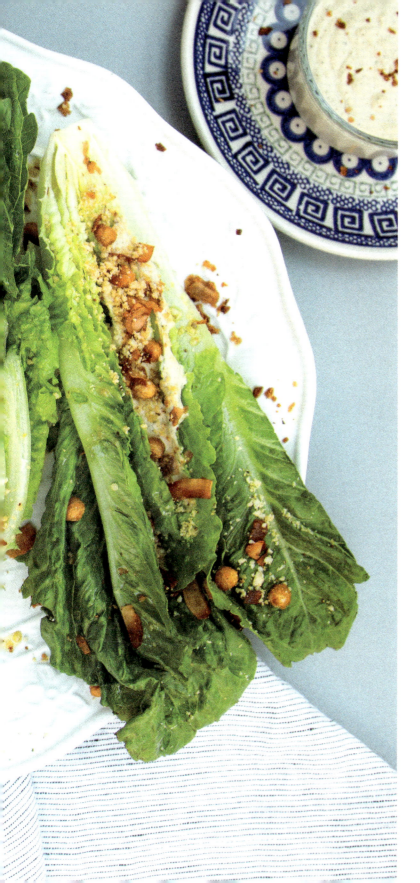

SALADS

I love salad. Always have, always will. And I'm not alone on this....salads are gracing the menus of almost every restaurant in the world, and that's not changing any time soon! They are nutritious, versatile, and a great way to enjoy a variety of vegetables. That said, there are lots of hidden calories and unnecessary ingredients in many salad dressings, and salad toppings. Many times, salads disguise themselves as "healthy", but in reality, they aren't as healthy as you'd like to think. I am determined to change that. . . at least in this cookbook. The salads at Choice are so full of flavor and nutrition. I've included some of our most loved salads, along with some of my personal favorites. These salads are just as delicious as they are nutritious.

CAESAR WEDGE with BRAZIL NUT "PARMESAN" & COCONUT "BAKON"

CAESAR WEDGE

INGREDIENTS:

¼ CUP
Brazil Nut "Parmesan"
(SEE RECIPE BELOW)

2
Romaine Hearts,
halved lengthwise

½ CUP
Caesar Dressing
(SEE RECIPE ON PG. 196)

¼ CUP
Coconut "Bakon"
(SEE RECIPE ON PG. 206)

½ CUP
Chickpea Croutons
(SEE RECIPE TO THE RIGHT)

PREPARATION:

01. Drizzle romaine halves with Caesar Dressing. Top with Brazil nut "Parmesan", Chickpea Croutons and Coconut "Bakon."

BRAZIL NUT "PARMESAN"

INGREDIENTS:
THIS RECIPE ALSO APPEARS ON PG. 208

½ CUP
Raw Brazil Nuts

3 TBSP
Raw Cashews

3 TBSP
Raw Hemp Seeds

1 TBSP
Nutritional Yeast

½ TSP
Himalayan Salt

¾ TBSP
Garlic Powder

PREPARATION:

01. Combine Brazil nuts, cashews and hemp seeds in a blender or food processor. Pulse until a sandy texture is achieved. Be careful! Pulsing too much can result in a Brazil nut butter!

02. Add the remaining ingredients into the blender and pulse again until you have a parmesan-like consistency. Again, be careful not to over blend.

03. Store in an airtight container for up to 2 weeks.

CHICKPEA CROUTONS

INGREDIENTS:

1 15 OZ. CAN
Chickpeas
(rinsed and dried)

1 TBSP
Olive Oil

1 TSP
Nutritional Yeast

½ TSP
Garlic Powder

½ TSP
Himalayan Salt

½ TSP
Onion Powder

⅛ TSP
Cayenne Pepper

PREPARATION:

01. Preheat the oven to 400°F.

02. Rinse the chickpeas and pat dry.

03. Combine the chickpeas with the remaining ingredients in a mixing bowl until all ingredients are evenly dispersed.

04. Bake in the oven until golden brown (Approximately 15 min.)

05. Store in an airtight container for approximately 4-5 days.

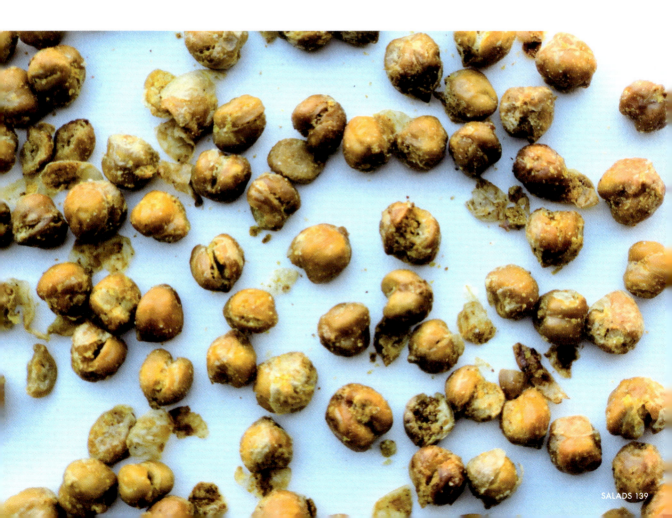

CRUNCHY CASHEW QUINOA THAI SALAD

Thai food is one of my favorite cuisines. Traditionally, the dishes are prepared with a lot of oil, salt and other heavy ingredients. This salad satisfies my Thai cravings, but in the form of a light and healthy meal.

INGREDIENTS:

2 CUPS
Cooked Quinoa (prepared according to package instructions)

2 CUPS
Red Cabbage, shredded (add more for extra crunch)

1 SMALL
Red Bell Pepper, diced

¼ CUP
Red Onion, diced

1 CUP
Carrots, shredded

½ CUP
Cilantro, chopped

¼ CUP
Green Onions, sliced

½ CUP
Cashew Halves (raw or roasted depending on your preference)

1 CUP
Edamame

Fresh Lime for Garnish

½ - 1 CUPS
Pad Thai Sauce
(SEE RECIPE ON PG. 205)

PREPARATION:

01. Add as much (or as little) Pad Thai Sauce as you'd like to the quinoa. I like to start with a little bit of dressing and usually add more to suit my taste preferences. Alternatively, you can save the dressing for later and add more when you are ready to eat. However, the flavors of the dressing usually soak into the salad so I like to add it to the quinoa first but that is totally up to you.

02. Next, fold in red bell pepper, red onion, cabbage, edamame and carrots into the quinoa. Garnish with cashews, cilantro and green onions.

03. Serve chilled or at room temperature with lime wedges, if desired.

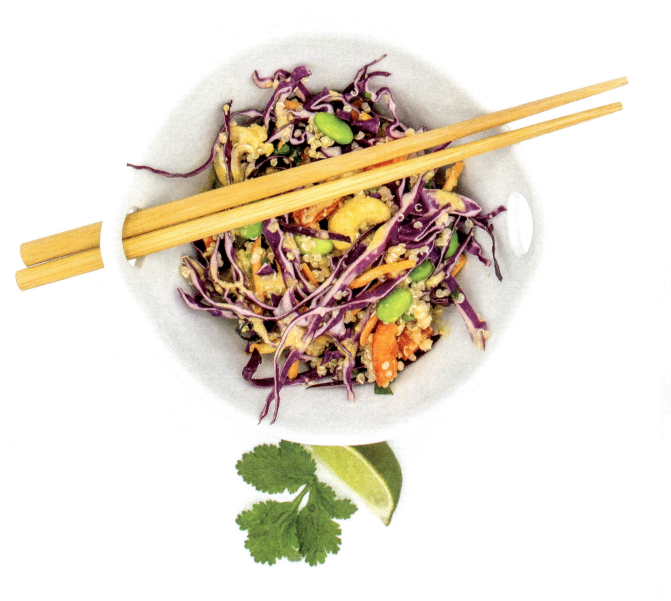

BBQ BLACK BEAN SALAD

This salad is one of my absolute favorites. I love to make the Cashew Ranch Dressing and BBQ Sauce and I always have them on hand. There are so many great things you can do with both. This is just a quick and delicious salad option with a ton of flavor. When I make this for dinner, I usually make some loaded baked potatoes to go with it, and my kiddos go crazy (in a good way). The BBQ sauce is a tad on the spicy side, but you can adjust that if you'd like.

NOTE:
The combination of the Cashew Ranch Dressing, and BBQ sauce helps mellow out the spice in this salad.

INGREDIENTS:

¼ CUP
BBQ Sauce
(SEE RECIPE ON PG. 200)

¼ CUP
Cashew Ranch Dressing
(SEE RECIPE ON PG. 198)

¼ CUP
Corn, steamed

2 CUPS
Black Beans, prepared
(SEE RECIPE TO THE RIGHT)

2 HEADS
Romaine, rinsed and chopped

1 CUP
Tomato, diced

¼ CUP
Red Onion, diced

2 LARGE
Avocados, diced and salted

PREPARATION:

01. Place your chopped romaine in a bowl, and top with rows of each item: corn, beans, tomatoes, onion and avocados.

02. Drizzle with BBQ Sauce and Cashew Ranch Dressing.

BLACK BEANS
INGREDIENTS:

1 15 OZ. CAN
Black Beans

1 TBSP
Olive Oil

½ TSP
Himalayan Salt

½ TSP
Garlic Powder

½ TSP
Onion Powder

PREPARATION

01. Rinse and drain 1 15 oz can black beans.

02. Heat 1 Tbsp of olive oil in a small saucepan over medium heat. Add Himalayan salt, garlic powder, onion powder and black beans, and cook until black beans are hot.

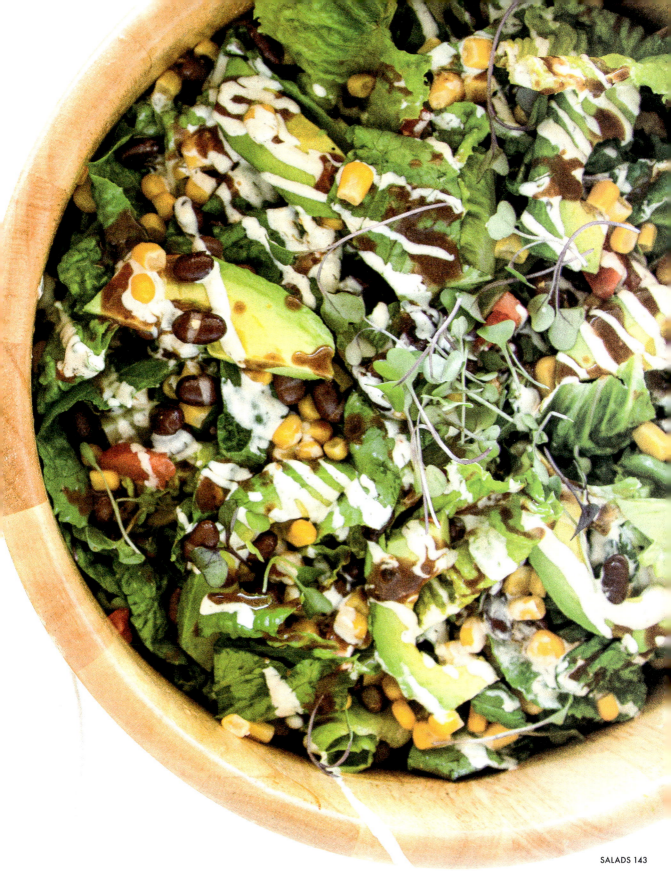

CHICKPEA SPINACH BUDDHA BOWL with LEMON GARLIC TAHINI DRESSING

This salad is just as colorful as it is tasty. It's loaded with protein, vitamin C, healthy fats, fiber, and minerals such as calcium, magnesium, and iron. The Lemon Garlic Tahini Dressing is the belle of the ball in this recipe. Among its many benefits, tahini contains more protein than milk and most nuts. It's a rich source of B vitamins, which can boost energy and brain function, and vitamin E, which is protective against heart disease and stroke.

MARINATED CHICKPEAS
INGREDIENTS:

- **2 15 OZ. CANS** Chickpeas, rinsed and drained *(SEE NOTE)*
- **1/2 MEDIUM** Lemon, juiced (about 3 tablespoons)
- **1 TBSP** Nutritional Yeast
- **1/2 TSP** Himalayan Salt (or to taste)
- **1/4 TSP** Garlic Powder
- **1 TBSP** Olive Oil
- **PINCH OF** Black Pepper

PREPARATION:

01. Drain and rinse chickpeas. Combine all ingredients and marinate chickpeas in the refrigerator for a minimum of 20 mins.

BUDDHA BOWL
INGREDIENTS:

- Marinated Chickpeas *(SEE RECIPE ABOVE)*
- **4-6 CUPS** Baby Spinach
- **1 MEDIUM** Red Bell Pepper, diced
- **1 LARGE** Avocado, diced and salted
- Lemon Garlic Tahini Dressing *(SEE RECIPE ON PG. 194)*
- **1 CUP** Cooked Quinoa *(PREPARE ACCORDING TO PACKAGE DIRECTIONS)*

PREPARATION:

01. Divide spinach between four bowls. Place ¼ cup of the cooked quinoa on top of the spinach (you can prepare quinoa in advance and serve cold, but I prefer to make the quinoa while I'm prepping everything else because I love the warm quinoa in this bowl).

02. Divide Marinated Chickpeas between your bowls, and sprinkle with bell pepper, and avocado.

03. Drizzle the Buddha bowl with Lemon Garlic Tahini dressing and serve immediately.

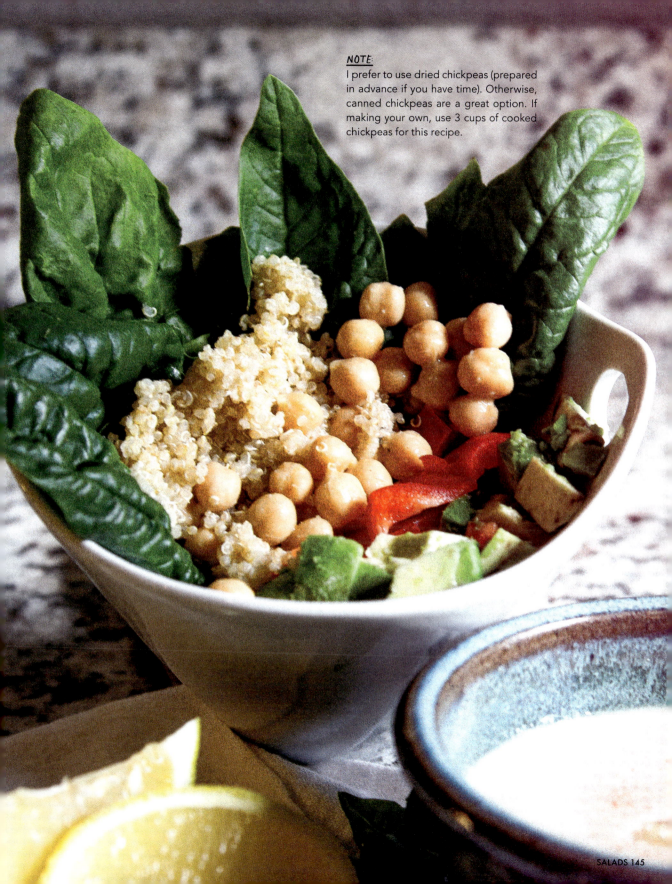

NOTE:
I prefer to use dried chickpeas (prepared in advance if you have time). Otherwise, canned chickpeas are a great option. If making your own, use 3 cups of cooked chickpeas for this recipe.

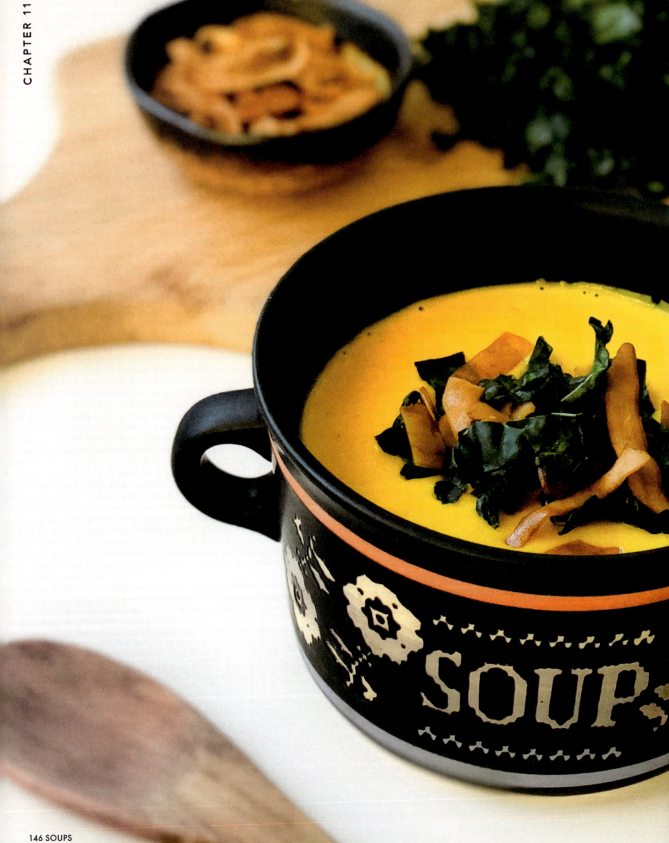

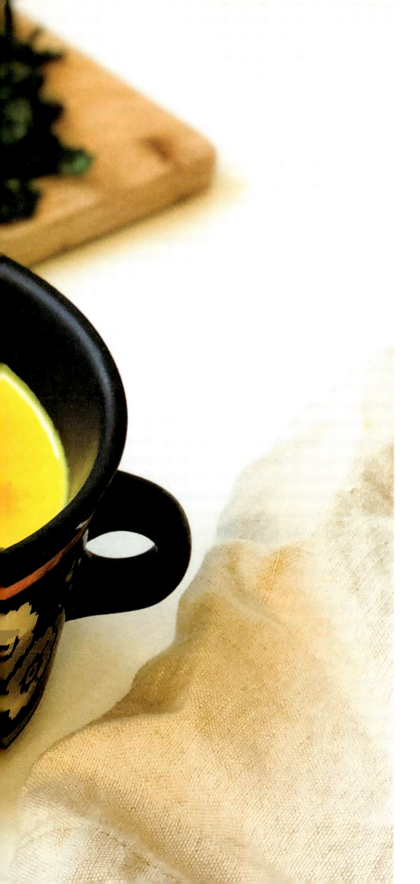

SOUPS

I love making soup in the colder seasons but let's be honest, I live in San Diego and the cold seasons are pretty few and far between (not that I'm complaining about it!). When those cold days do arrive, eating or drinking something hot increases the sensation of being warm and helps boost my mood. You may have heard about SAD (seasonal affective disorder), also known as "Winter Depression". This is caused by lack of sunlight (and thus, vitamin D) due to cold weather. People experiencing this often crave carbohydrate-rich foods and report feeling better during or after consumption. Rather than reaching for the cake, chips, or cookies, I opt for healthier options with complex carbohydrates. Here are a few of my favorite soup recipes with complex carbs (amongst other incredible nutrients) to warm up with on those cold winter days.

BROCCOLI SOUP
MAKES: 4 CUPS

I'm so excited to share this Choice favorite with you. This soup is made creamy with cashews and avocado. It's full of nutrition and it just so happens to be one of my favorite things to eat on our café menu during the fall and winter months!

INGREDIENTS:

2 1/3 CUPS
Water

1/2 CUP
Raw Cashews, soaked

1 CUP
Broccoli
(¼ cup chopped florets, reserved)

1/2
Avocado

1/2 CLOVE
Garlic

1 TBSP
Olive Oil

1 1/2 TBSP
Lemon Juice

2 1/2 TBSP
Nutritional Yeast

1 TSP
Agave

3/4 TSP
Onion Powder

2 1/2 TSP
Himalayan Salt

1/8 TSP
Cumin

1 TSP
Black Pepper

PREPARATION:

01. Add all ingredients (except ¼ cup of broccoli florets) to your high powered blender and blend on high until smooth (about 5 minutes).

02. Add florets and blend on medium for an additional 30 seconds, or until desired consistency is achieved.

03. Heat and serve. Can also be enjoyed chilled.

NOTE:
Any leftovers can be stored in the fridge for up to 5 days.

BONUS OPTION: I love enjoying this soup with the addition of some Coconut "Bakon," massaged kale, and cooked quinoa. It's also great on its own! *(SEE RECIPE FOR COCONUT "BAKON" ON PG. 206)*

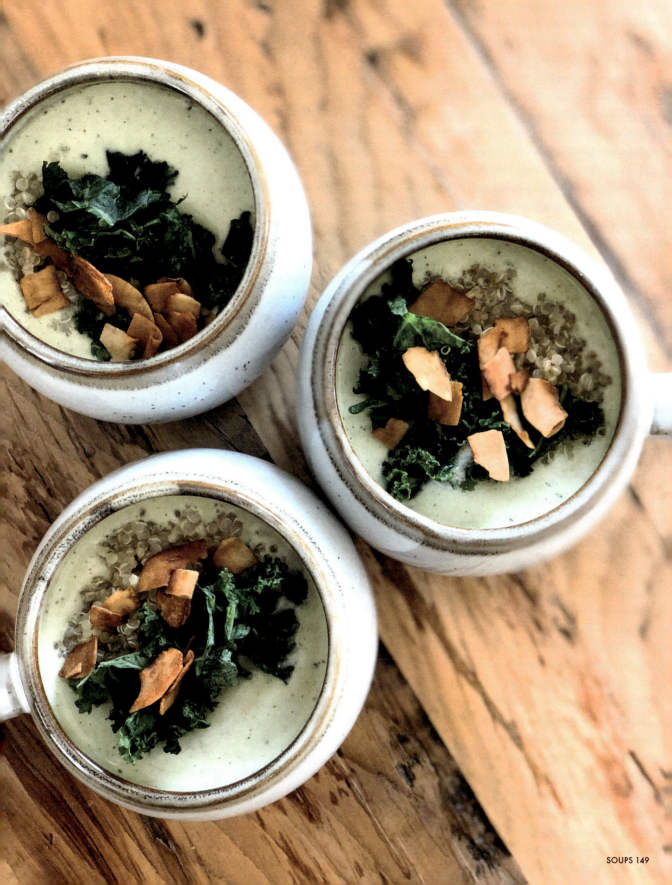

"CHEESY" CAULIFLOWER SOUP with MASSAGED KALE & COCONUT "BAKON"

MAKES: 4 CUPS

INGREDIENTS:

1 LARGE
Cauliflower, cut into small florets

1
Carrot, diced

1 TBSP
Olive Oil

1 SMALL
Yellow Onion, diced

3 CLOVES
Garlic, minced

3 MEDIUM
Golden Potatoes, cut into 1" cubes

3/4 CUP
Raw Cashews, soaked for 20 mins in warm water

3 CUBES
Veggie Bouillon

6 CUPS
Water + more to thin out as desired

1/4 CUP
Nutritional Yeast

6 SPRIGS
Fresh Thyme

1
Bay Leaf

1 1/2 TSP
Turmeric

1 1/2 TSP
Ground Ginger

1/4 TSP
Himalayan Salt
(+ more to taste)

1 TSP
Onion Powder

1 TBSP
Lemon Juice

4 TBSP
Coconut "Bakon"

1 CUP
Curly Kale, massaged

1/2 TSP
Garlic Powder

PREPARATION:

01. In a large pot over medium heat, add olive oil, diced onion and salt. Sauté for a few minutes, until onions are translucent.

02. Add the diced carrot and cook for about 5 minutes, until carrots are softened.

03. Add the fresh garlic, cauliflower, potatoes, cashews, thyme and bay leaf and toss everything to coat.

04. Pour in the water and veggie bouillon and bring to a simmer. Stir in the nutritional yeast, turmeric, ginger, onion powder, garlic powder, and lemon juice and cook for about 15 to 20 minutes, or until all vegetables are soft. Discard bay leaf and thyme sprigs.

05. In small batches, transfer to a high powered blender and purée until silky smooth. Top with massaged kale and Coconut "Bakon".

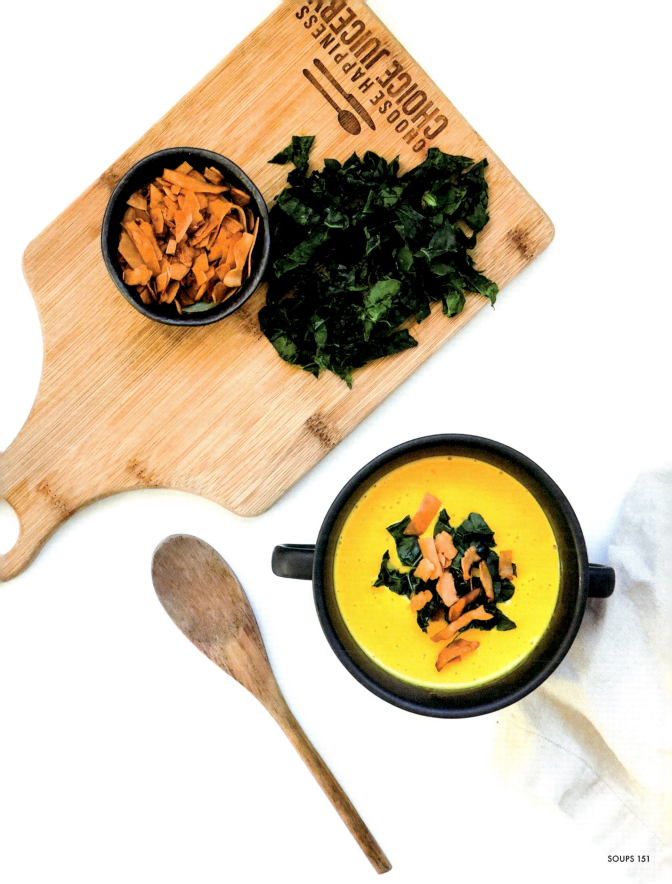

TORTILLA SOUP with OYSTER MUSHROOM SHREDDED "CHICKEN"

OYSTER MUSHROOM SHREDDED "CHICKEN"
INGREDIENTS:

1 LB.
Oyster Mushrooms, shredded
(simply pull apart by hand into small shreds)

2 TBSP
Olive Oil

1/2 TSP
Cumin

1/2 TSP
Ancho Chilli Powder

1/2 TSP
Garlic, minced

1/8 TSP
Oregano

1/2 TSP
Coriander

1/2 TSP
Onion Powder

TORTILLA SOUP
INGREDIENTS:

3 TBSP
Olive Oil

1/2 SMALL
White Onion, diced

2 CLOVES
Garlic, minced

1-2 SMALL
Chipotle Peppers in Adobo Sauce, coarsely chopped
(use more or less to achieve desired spice)

1/2 TSP
Himalayan Salt
(+ more to taste)

2 TSP
Ground Cumin

3 CUBES
Veggie Bouillon
(I love Edward and Sons "Not-Chick'n" Bouillon Cubes but you can use any vegetable broth if you can't find this brand)

5 CUPS
Water

1 1/2 CUP
Oyster Mushroom Shredded "Chicken"

1/2 TSP
Garlic Powder

1/2 TSP
Onion Powder

2 TBSP
Nutritional Yeast

FOR SERVING:

5 SMALL
Organic Corn Tortillas
(or use tortilla chips)

2-3 TBSP
Olive Oil (if using tortillas)

1/2 TSP
Himalayan Salt

1/4 TSP
Paprika

4-6
Lime Wedges

1/4 CUP
Cilantro, chopped

1 LARGE
Avocado, diced and salted

1/4 CUP
Brazil Nut "Parmesan"
(SEE RECIPE ON PG. 208)

OYSTER MUSHROOM SHREDDED "CHICKEN"
PREPARATION:

01. Rub oil and spices onto shredded mushrooms and roast at 400° F for 35 mins, making sure to turn every few minutes so they don't get too crispy or charred.

TORTILLA SOUP
PREPARATION:

01. Heat olive oil in a large pot over medium heat. Once hot, add diced onion and minced garlic. Sauté, stirring occasionally for 3-5 minutes or until onions are translucent.

02. Add chipotle peppers, Himalayan salt, garlic powder, onion powder, nutritional yeast and cumin. Sauté, stirring frequently, for 3-4 more minutes.

03. Add the bouillon cubes and water and bring to a low boil. Then reduce heat and simmer for at least 15 minutes (up to 30 minutes).

04. Once the oyster mushroom shredded "chicken" is done, add it to the pot. Taste and adjust spices as needed.

05. In the meantime, if you're using tortillas - preheat the oven to 380° F. Cut corn tortillas into bite-sized strips, drizzle with 2-3 Tbsp of olive oil or avocado oil, and toss in paprika and ½ tsp Himalayan salt, to coat. Arrange in a single layer on a sheet tray and bake for 10-15 minutes or until they are golden brown. Watch carefully toward the end or they can burn! (if using tortilla chips, you can skip this step)

06. To serve, place tortilla strips or chips in serving bowls, top with soup, and garnish with avocado, cilantro, lime wedges and Brazil Nut "Parmesan".

TUSCAN WHITE BEAN & KALE SOUP

Okay, so this book was almost done. Like, already in the hands of my editor (done) when I made this soup one night for my family on a whim. I was inspired to make a Tuscan soup after hearing all about a girlfriend's trip to Italy earlier in the week. It also happened to be the first week of cold weather in San Diego (I realize I run this risk of being ridiculed by calling San Diego cold, but in my defense, it was a drastic drop of about 25 degrees).

I wanted a soup, but I was not in the mood for my go-to's and feeling the Italian inspiration, I decided to whip up this Tuscan inspired white bean soup with some veggies from the garden. I happened to have more kale than I knew what to do with, and this recipe was the perfect way to use it up. I don't always hit a home run on my first attempt, but WOW was I pleased with this one (as were all three of my kiddos). Now, it's rare to have all three on the same page, but when that happens I know it's a recipe worth sharing, so here it is!

INGREDIENTS:

2 15 OZ. CANS
Cannellini Beans, rinsed and drained

1 SMALL BUNCH OF
Dino Kale, ribs removed, chopped and massaged

1 MEDIUM
White Onion, diced

1 CUP
Carrots, peeled and diced

4 CLOVES
Garlic, grated

1 SMALL SPRIG
Rosemary, leaves removed and chopped
(roughly 1 tsp + more to taste)

1 MEDIUM
Lemon, juiced

1/4 CUP
Nutritional Yeast

1/2 TSP
Onion Powder

1/2 TSP
Garlic Powder

1/4 TSP
Black Pepper
(+ more to taste)

3 TBSP
Olive Oil, (the very best you can get your hands on - this makes a huge difference) + more to drizzle

3 CUBES
Veggie Bouillon
(I love Edward and Sons "Not-Chick'n" Bouillon Cubes but you can use any vegetable broth if you can't find this brand)

2 LARGE
Tomatoes, diced

1 TSP
Red Pepper Flakes (omit if you don't like it spicy)

6 CUPS
Water
(+ more for boiling potatoes)

2 SMALL
Potatoes, peeled, diced and boiled in a separate pot until softened
(FORK SHOULD GO THROUGH EASILY)

1/4 CUP
Italian Parsley, chopped

1/4 CUP
Brazil Nut "Parmesan"
(OPTIONAL SEE RECIPE ON PG. 208)

1/2 TSP
Himalayan Salt
(+ more to taste)

PREPARATION:

01. In a small pot, boil water + 1 tsp of salt. Toss in diced potatoes and boil until tender. Drain and set aside.

02. In a large, heavy-bottom pot or dutch oven, heat olive oil over medium heat. Add diced onions and saute 6-8 minutes, until translucent.

03. Lower heat to medium-low and add the carrots and garlic, Himalayan salt, black pepper and chili flakes (if using), and cook another 7- 9 minutes until vegetables are tender.

04. Add the tomatoes, dino kale and lemon juice, and continue sautéing, stirring occasionally, for 7-8 minutes.

05. Add in veggie bouillon, water, cannellini beans, boiled potatoes, garlic powder, onion powder, rosemary, black pepper, and nutritional yeast.

06. Bring to soup to boil, turn heat down and simmer for 15 minutes.

07. Stir in fresh Italian parsley. Adjust salt and seasoning to your taste, ladle into bowls, and top each with a sprinkling of Brazil Nut "Parmesan".

08. Serve immediately, with some gluten-free bread

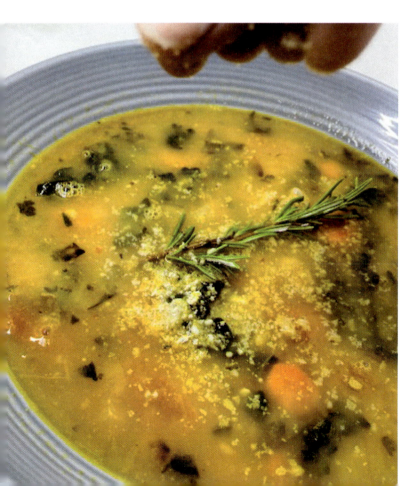

BENEFITS:

Cannellini beans, which are also called *white kidney beans*, are a nutritional powerhouse! They're packed with fiber and protein and are a good source of numerous micronutrients, including folate, magnesium, and vitamin B6. White Kidney Beans are also rich in copper and iron.

Copper primarily aids energy production and iron metabolism, while folate is utilized in DNA synthesis. Iron has numerous important functions, including producing hemoglobin, which transports oxygen throughout your body.

What's more, white beans are high in polyphenol antioxidants, which combat oxidative stress in your body. In turn, this may protect you against chronic illnesses, including heart disease and certain cancers.

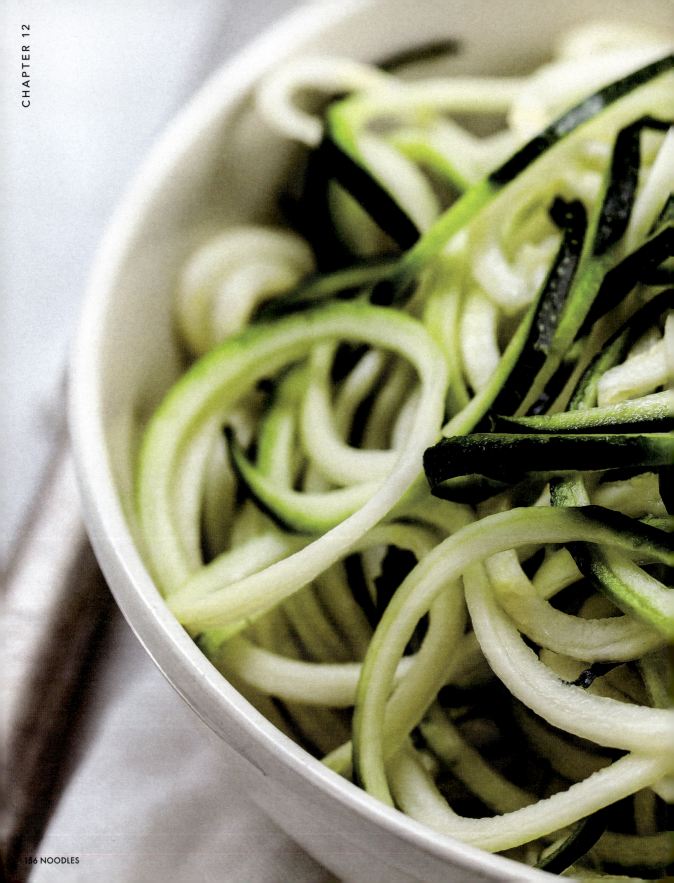

CHAPTER 12

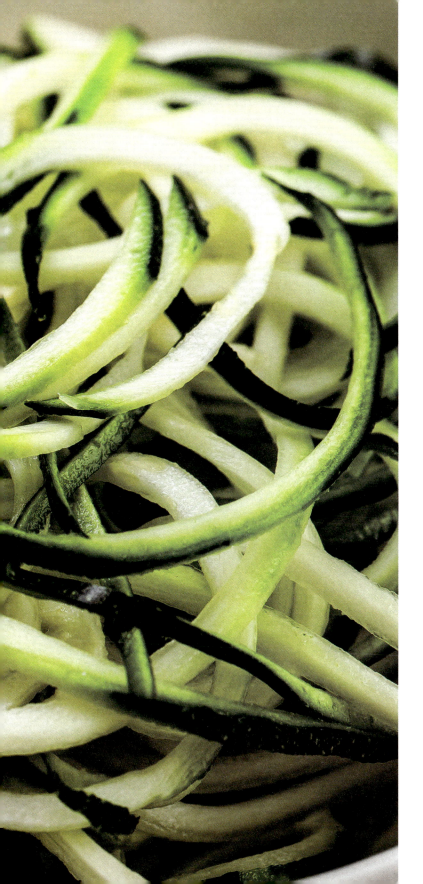

NOODLES

Fortunately, gluten-free noodles are widely available these days. While I love amazing pasta noodles, pasta (even gluten-free pasta) can be heavy to eat, so I enjoy having pasta-like dishes with noodle alternatives as an option. In fact, this chapter should have been called "noodle alternatives," because that's really what these recipes are! Enjoy!

"ALFREDO" ZOODLE PASTA

INGREDIENTS:

6 LARGE
Zucchinis, spiralized
(use spiralizer to make zoodles - available online)

2 LARGE
Portobello Mushrooms, stems removed

2 TBSP
Brazil Nut "Parmesan"
(SEE RECIPE ON PG. 208)

1 CUP
"Alfredo" Sauce, warmed
(SEE RECIPE ON PG. 199)

2 TBSP
Olive Oil

1/8 TSP
Himalayan Salt

1/4 TSP
Garlic Powder

PREPARATION:

01. Preheat the oven to 375°F.

02. Prepare the portobello mushrooms by removing the stems and cutting them into ¼ inch slices. Toss in a bowl with 1 Tbsp olive oil and sprinkle with salt and garlic powder.

03. Lay mushrooms onto a roasting pan and roast in the oven for 20-30 mins.

04. Meanwhile, 'zoodle' your zucchinis (turning them into zucchini noodles), toss them in 1 Tbsp olive oil (more if desired) and sprinkle with salt. Zoodles can be lightly sauteed in a pan, or enjoyed raw.

05. When zoodles are ready, toss with "Alfredo" Sauce, and place roasted mushrooms on top before sprinkling with Brazil Nut "Parmesan".

NOTE:
You can interchange the zucchini for yams or gluten free noodles. This is such a fun and easy recipe, and an amazing way to pack in the veggies (when using zucchini or yams).

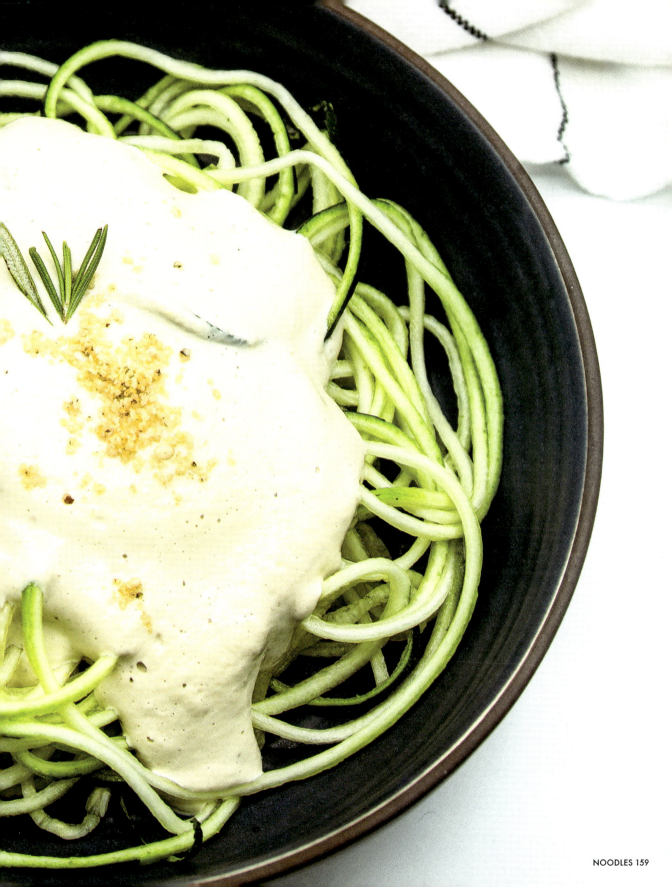

KELP NOODLES (A GREAT BASE FOR DIFFERENT PASTA SAUCES)

Kelp Noodles are an amazing low-calorie, low-carb, fat-free, sugar-free, nutrient-dense food! Full of vitamins A, B, and C as well as minerals like magnesium, calcium, zinc and iron.

Kelp noodles also fit into a range of diets. They contain only water, kelp, and sodium alginate (a naturally occurring salt in brown seaweed). As a result, kelp noodles are gluten-free, vegan, and free of all common allergens.

INGREDIENTS:

1 BAG OF
Kelp Noodles

BOWL OF
Water

¼ CUP
Lemon Juice

1 TBSP
Himalayan Salt

PREPARATION:

01. Open the bag of kelp noodles and drain the liquid.

02. Cut noodles into quarters using kitchen scissors. Place in a bowl and cover with water.

03. Add ¼ cup lemon juice and 1 Tbsp salt. Soak for an hour. Note: If you skip this step, the noodles will be chewy and less enjoyable. The texture is way more enjoyable when soaked. Plus, soaking the noodles prepares them for taking on extra flavor from the sauce.

04. Add whatever sauce or toppings you want to complete this simple (and YUMMY) dish.

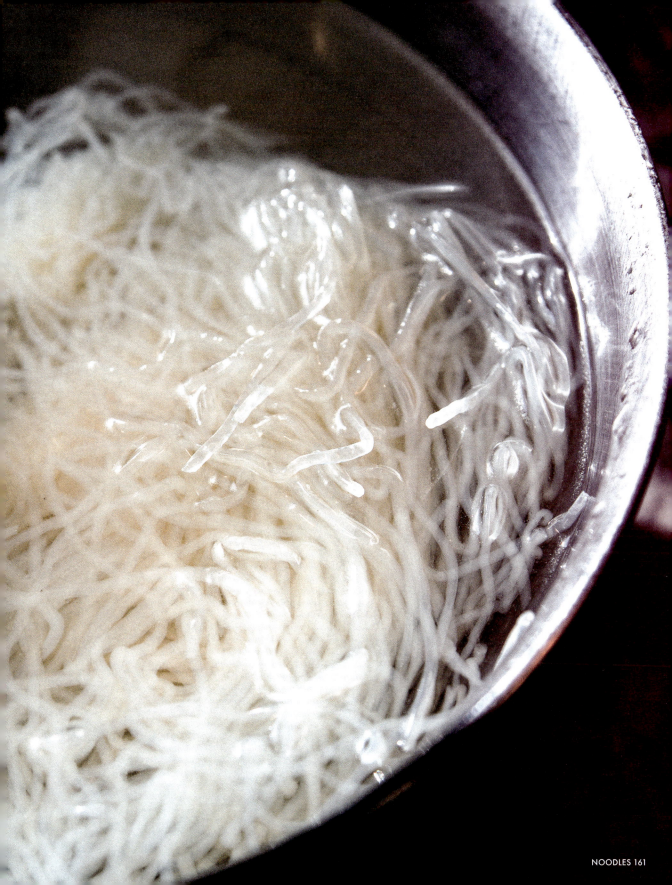

KELP NOODLE PAD THAI (SERVES 2)

INGREDIENTS:

1 PACKAGE
Kelp Noodles
(FOLLOW PREP INSTRUCTIONS ON PG. 160)

1 CUP
Red Bell Pepper, thinly sliced

1 CUP
Carrot, grated or thinly sliced

1 CUP
Curly Kale, ribs removed, massaged (about 3 min), and torn into small pieces

1 TBSP
Basil, chopped

1 TBSP
Cilantro, chopped

1 TBSP
Green Onion, sliced

2 TBSP
Almonds, roasted and chopped

1 CUP
Pad Thai Sauce
(SEE RECIPE ON PG. 205)

PREPARATION:

01. Place prepared kelp noodles (prep instructions can be found on pg. 160) in a bowl, toss in red bell pepper, carrot, massaged curly kale, basil, cilantro and green onion.

02. Add Pad Thai sauce and mix well.

03. Top with roasted almonds and serve immediately.

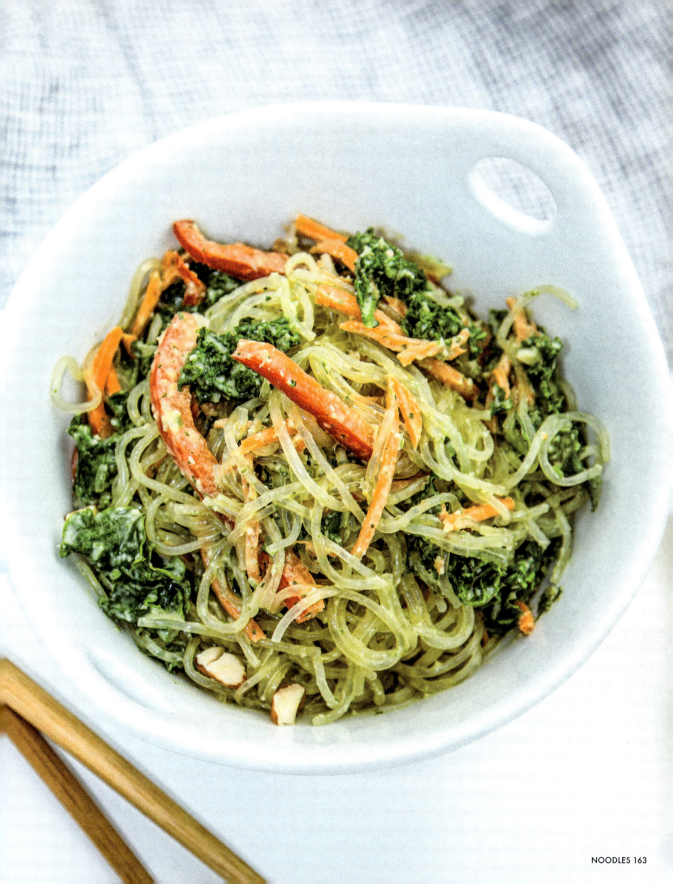

SUN DRIED TOMATO KELP NOODLE PASTA (SERVES 2)

INGREDIENTS:

1 PACKAGE
Kelp Noodles
(FOLLOW PREP INSTRUCTIONS ON PG. 160)

1 ½ CUPS
Arugula

1 CUP
Sun Dried Tomato Pesto
(SEE RECIPE ON PG. 202)

2 TBSP
Capers

PREPARATION:

01. Place prepared kelp noodles (prep instructions can be found on pg. 160) in a large bowl.

02. Add arugula and Sun Dried Tomato Pesto. Mix until well combined.

03. Divide between two dishes and sprinkle with capers

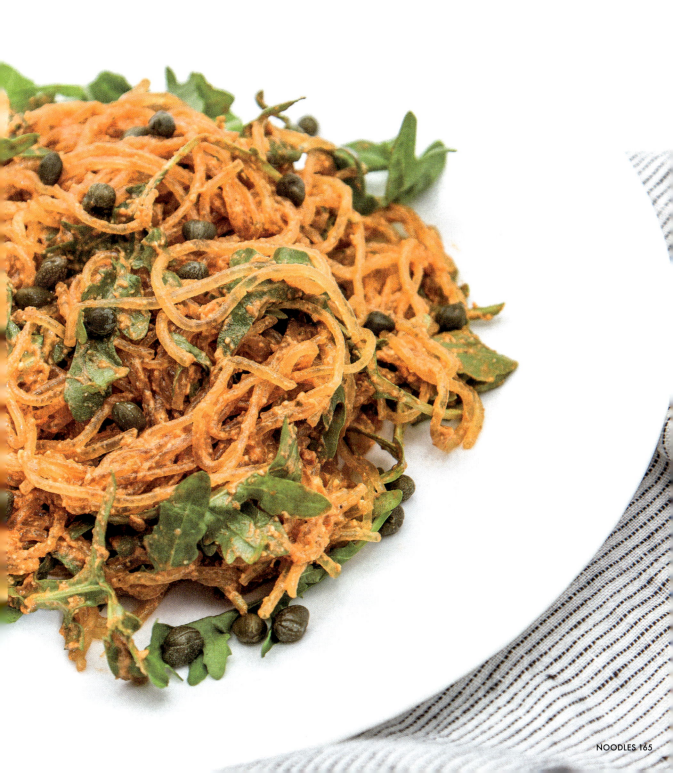

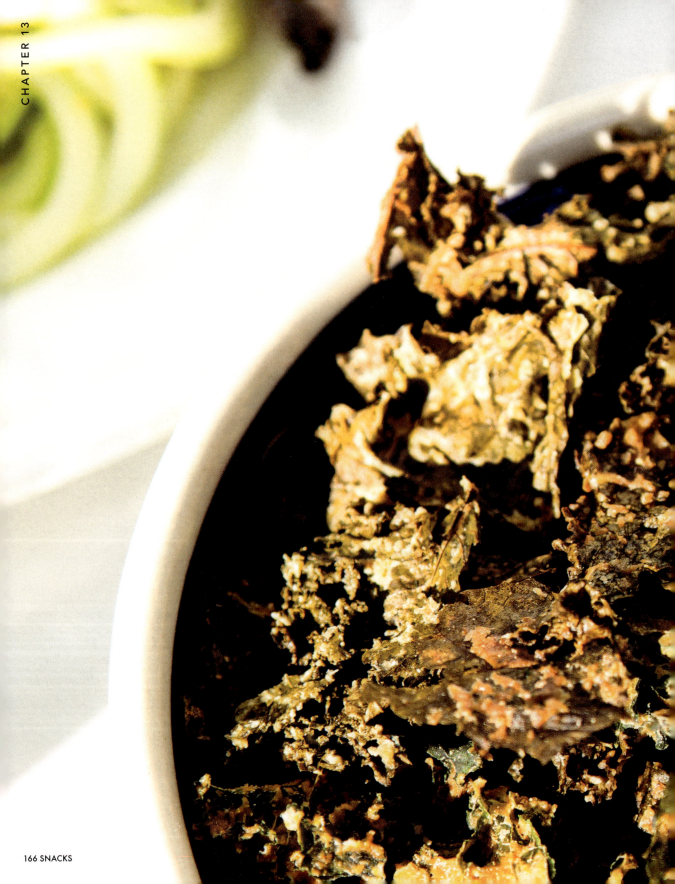

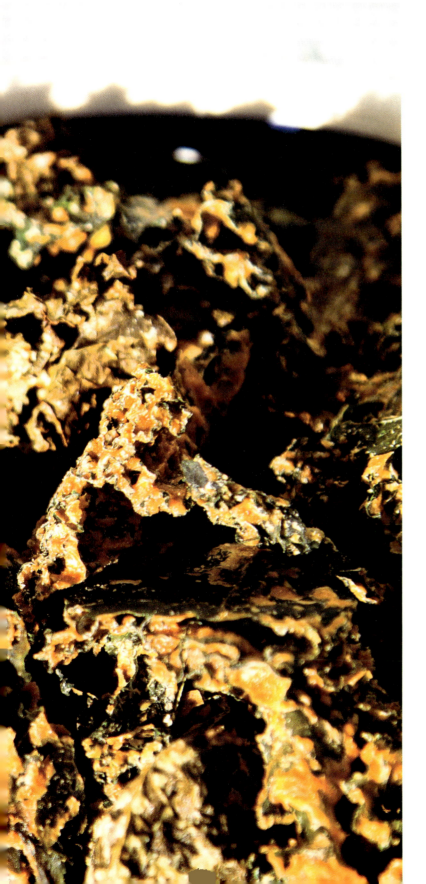

SNACKS

One of the best ways to make healthy choices is to have healthy choices easily accessible. I often get so busy that I skip hungry and go straight to starving! Not ideal. When I'm in that "hangry" mode, I am way less likely to make healthy choices if they aren't convenient. So keeping healthy snacks around helps to ensure I'm making healthy food choices. Chips are always an easy go to, but traditional chips often have little to no nutritional value and are packed with unhealthy fatty oils and way too much salt, along with preservatives and additives. Kale chips are a much healthier choice! They have the same yummy crunch with a healthy dose of flavor and nutrition.

CHIPOTLE KALE CHIPS

The perfect blend of smokey and spicy, these kale chips are sure to curb your cravings for their unhealthy counterparts.

INGREDIENTS:

5 CUPS
Curly Kale, packed with ribs removed

1 CUP (OR MORE)
Chipotle "Cheese" Sauce
(SEE RECIPE ON PG. 192)

PREPARATION:

01. Preheat the oven to 250°F.

02. Wash the kale, then carefully dry the leaves.

03. Strip and discard the leaves from the stems and place into a bowl, roughly tearing any large pieces.

04. Pour the Chipotle "Cheese" Sauce on top of the kale.

05. Using clean hands, massage the mixture into the kale for 1 minute to evenly coat the leaves.

06. Line two baking sheets with parchment paper, then spread the kale chips over the sheets, as evenly and as possible, to ensure even cooking time.

07. Bake between 1 ½ - 2 hours (time varies according to the dryness of the kale), tossing halfway through the baking, until the kale has dried out and is crispy (but not burnt). Keep a close eye on the kale at the end of the cooking process, and remove any edges that look too dark.

08. Enjoy immediately or keep in an airtight container for up to 1 week.

NOTE:
These are best made in a dehydrator. However, the method above works great, too. If you have a dehydrator, dehydrate the Kale Chips at 115°F for about 8 to 10 hours, or until dry and crispy.

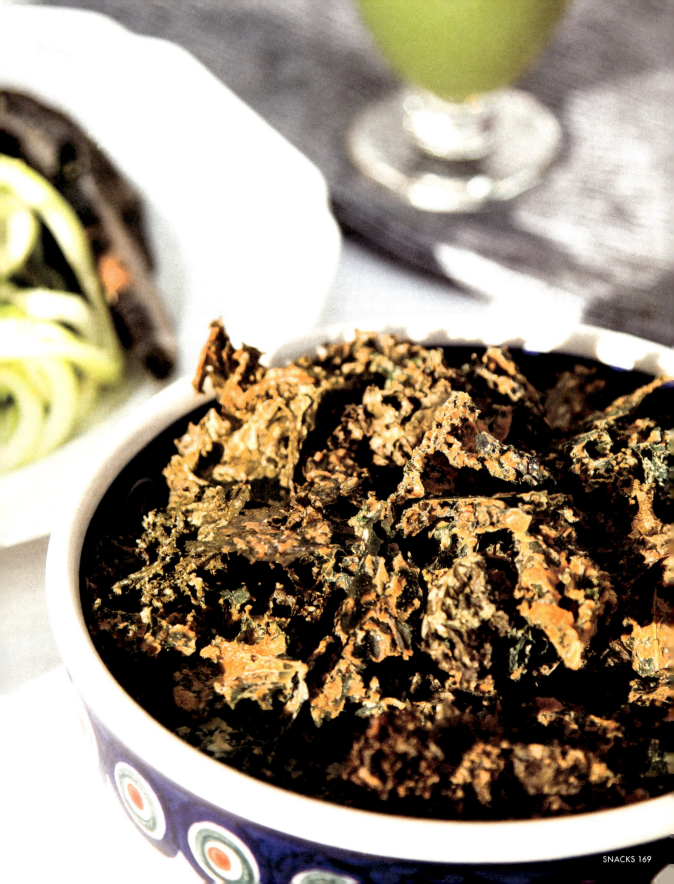

SNACKS 169

RANCH KALE CHIPS

These kale chips fly off the shelves at Choice - and for good reason. The Ranch Dressing is unbelievably delicious, and the crunch of the kale will leave you wanting more with every bite. They are easy to make and they keep well in an airtight container for up to a week, making them the perfect snack to keep on hand for when those cravings kick up.

INGREDIENTS:

5 CUPS
Curly Kale, packed with ribs removed

1 CUP (OR MORE)
Cashew Ranch Dressing
(SEE RECIPE ON PG. 198)

PREPARATION:

01. Preheat the oven to 250°F.

02. Wash the kale, then carefully dry the leaves.

03. Strip and discard the leaves from the stems and place into a bowl, roughly tearing any large pieces.

04. Pour the Cashew Ranch Dressing on top of the kale.

05. Using clean hands, massage the mixture into the kale for 1 minute to evenly coat the leaves.

06. Line two baking sheets with parchment paper, then spread the kale chips over the sheets, as evenly as possible, to ensure even cooking time.

07. Bake between 1 ½ - 2 hours (time varies according to the dryness of the kale), tossing halfway through baking, until the kale has dried out and is crispy (but not burnt). Keep a close eye on the kale at the end of the cooking process, and remove any edges that look too dark.

08. Enjoy immediately or keep in an airtight container for up to 1 week.

NOTE:
These are best made in a dehydrator. However, the method above works great, too. If you have a dehydrator, dehydrate the Kale Chips at 115°F for about 8 to 10 hours, or until dry and crispy.

"SOUR CREAM" & ONION KALE CHIPS

I love sour cream and onion anything (vegan of course) so it's only natural that I would love "Sour Cream" & Onion Kale Chips. This is another great item to have around when you want to have a healthy little snack packed with a ton of flavor (and nutrition).

INGREDIENTS:

1 CUP
"Sour Cream" & Onion Dressing *(SEE RECIPE ON PG. 197)*

5 CUPS
Curly Kale, packed with ribs removed

PREPARATION:

01. Preheat the oven to 250°F.

02. Wash the kale, then carefully dry the leaves.

03. Strip and discard the leaves from the stems and place into a bowl, roughly tearing any large pieces.

04. Pour the "Sour Cream" & Onion Dressing on top of the kale.

05. Using clean hands, massage the mixture into the kale for 1 minute to evenly coat the leaves.

06. Line two baking sheets with parchment paper, then spread the kale chips over the sheets, as evenly and as possible, to ensure even cooking time.

07. Bake between 1 ½ - 2 hours (time varies according to the dryness of the kale), tossing halfway through baking, until the kale has dried out and is crispy (but not burnt). Keep a close eye on the kale at the end of the cooking process, and remove any edges that look too dark.

08. Enjoy immediately or keep in an airtight container for up to 1 week.

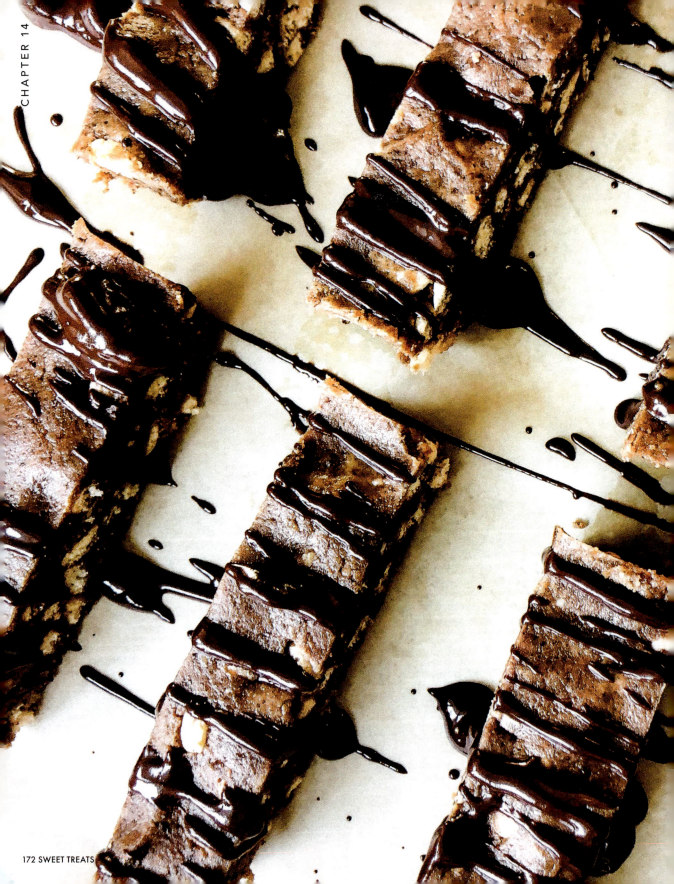

CHAPTER 14

172 SWEET TREATS

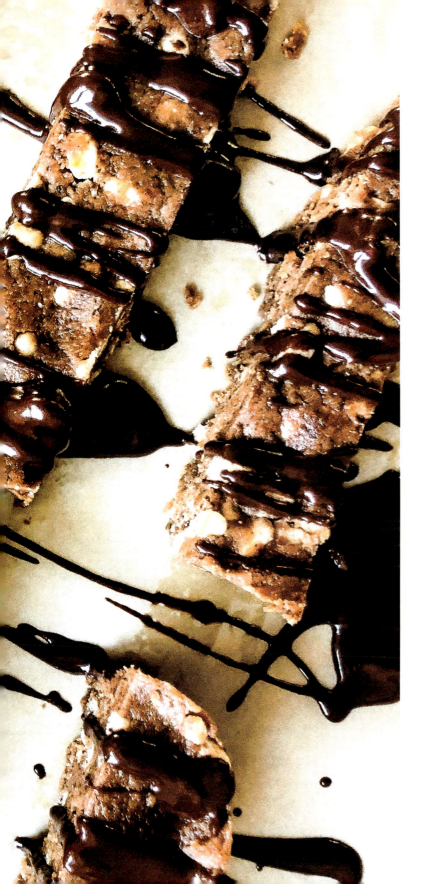

SWEET TREATS

Turns out that you can have your cake and eat it too! But seriously, satisfying your sweet tooth with healthier choices has never been easier. There are so many ways to satisfy your sweet cravings while also fueling yourself with powerful nutrients. Remember, the food we eat can either be the most powerful form of medicine, or the slowest form of poison. So when it comes to sweets, it's important to keep up those healthy choices.

CHOCOLATE CRISP PROTEIN BARS

These should come with a warning, "highly addictive". But hey, if you're going to eat habit-forming foods, these aren't a bad choice! Loaded with nutrition, sweetened naturally with whole dates and packed with protein, there isn't much more you could ask for out of a sweet treat.

INGREDIENTS:

10 LARGE
Mejool Dates, pitted

1 CUP
Almond Butter

2 TBSP
Raw Cacao Powder

1 TBSP
Coconut Oil, melted

PINCH
Cinnamon

¼ CUP
Choice Superfood Protein (available online or at any Choice location)

1 ¼ TSP
Pure Vanilla Extract

¼ TSP
Himalayan Salt

¾ CUP
Sprouted Brown Rice Crisps (usually found in cereal department, can be substituted for puffed quinoa)

CHOCOLATE DRIZZLE
OPTIONAL:

½ CUP
Vegan Chocolate Chips (SEE *NOTE*)

½ TSP
Coconut Oil

NOTE:
Melt ½ cup chocolate chips with ½ tsp coconut oil

PREPARATION:

01. Process all ingredients (except the sprouted brown rice crisps) in a food processor until well combined (you want a dough-like consistency).

02. Fold in the sprouted brown rice crisps and press protein bar dough into a greased 8" pan.

03. Place in the freezer for 10 minutes to harden a bit. If using the chocolate drizzle, use this time to melt your vegan chocolate chips with the additional coconut oil (set aside - used later in step 5).

04. Pull your 8" pan out of the freezer and cut your protein bars into rectangular squares (or whatever shape your heart desires) using a sharp knife. I like to cut around the edges and pop the whole thing out, then lay on a flat surface to cut out my bars. Do it however you prefer.

05. After your bars are cut, place them on a large serving plate lined with parchment paper and if using, drizzle the melted chocolate all over.

06. Place back in the freezer for 2 minutes. Move to an airtight container and store in the fridge for up to 2 weeks.

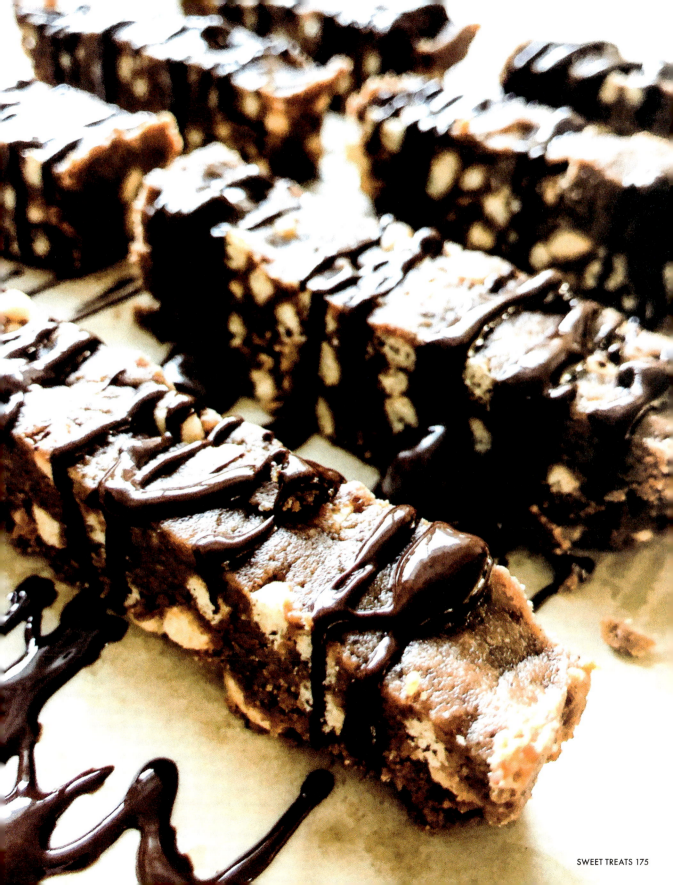

GLUTEN-FREE CHOCOLATE CHIP BANANA BREAD

One of the most popular items at Choice is our Chocolate Chip Banana Bread Muffins. This recipe is a variation of that beloved Choice treat. You would never believe this loaf is packed with our Choice Superfood Protein, gluten-free, and plant-based! This extra nutritious Chocolate Chip Banana Bread is sure to be a crowd pleaser!

NOTE:
This batter can be baked in muffin tins, for the BEST Gluten-Free Chocolate Chip Banana Bread muffins ever!

INGREDIENTS:

- 3/4 CUP Coconut Oil, melted
- 1/2 CUP Sprouted Vanilla Almond Milk
- 1 1/2 TSP Pure Vanilla Extract
- 1/2 CUP Coconut Sugar
- 2 TBSP Flaxseed Meal
- 1 CUP Buckwheat Flour
- 3/4 CUP Coconut Flour
- 1/2 CUP Almond Flour
- 3 TBSP Choice Superfood Protein (available in stores, or online)
- 1/4 TSP Baking Soda
- 1/8 TSP Baking Powder
- 1/2 TSP Himalayan Salt
- 2 CUPS Ripe Bananas, mashed
- 2 TBSP Coconut Flakes
- 1/2 CUP Vegan Chocolate Chips

PREPARATION:

01. Preheat the oven to 350°F. Line a loaf pan with parchment paper and set aside.

02. In a large bowl, add coconut oil, coconut sugar, Sprouted Vanilla Almond Milk, and vanilla and blend until incorporated.

03. In a separate medium sized bowl, add flaxseed meal, buckwheat flour, coconut flour, almond flour, Himalayan salt, baking powder, baking soda, and Choice Superfood Protein and mix well.

04. Add the mashed bananas to the bowl with coconut oil, coconut sugar, etc. and blend until thoroughly incorporated.

05. Add the dry ingredients to the bowl with the wet ingredients and mix to combine, then fold in the coconut flakes and vegan chocolate chips.

07. Bake for 30 minutes, or until a toothpick comes out clean. Edges should be slightly browned.

08. Allow the Gluten-Free Chocolate Chip Banana Bread to cool in the pan completely before slicing.

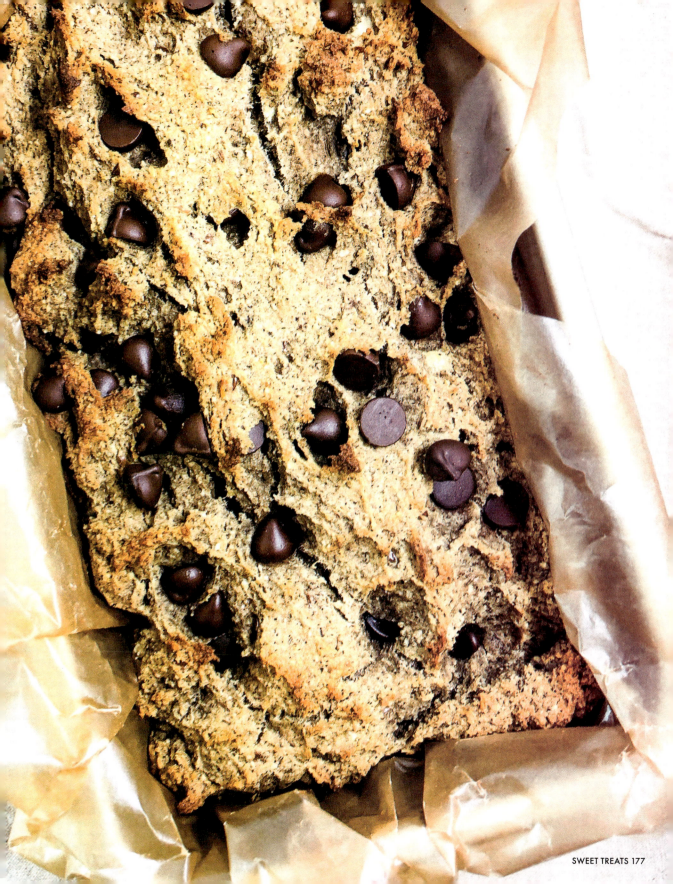

GLUTEN-FREE PUMPKIN LOAF

Similar to our famous seasonal Pumpkin Muffins at Choice, this Gluten-Free Pumpkin Loaf is vegan and totally delicious!

INGREDIENTS:

½ CUP
Coconut Oil, melted

½ CUP
Sprouted Vanilla Almond Milk

1 ½ TSP
Pure Vanilla Extract

½ CUP
Coconut Sugar

2 TBSP
Flaxseed Meal

1 CUP
Buckwheat Flour

6 OZ
Coconut Flour

½ CUP
Almond Flour

3 TBSP
Choice Superfood Protein
(available in stores, or online)

⅛ TSP
Baking Soda

¼ TSP
Baking Powder

½ TSP
Himalayan Salt

1 ½ CUPS
Pumpkin Purée

1 ½ TBSP
Pumpkin Spice
(SEE RECIPE BELOW)

NOTE:
Not all pumpkin spices taste the same. I highly encourage the use of this blend.

PREPARATION:

01. Preheat the oven to 350°F. Line a loaf pan with parchment paper and set aside.

02. In a large bowl, combine coconut oil, coconut sugar, Sprouted Vanilla Almond Milk, vanilla, and pumpkin purée and blend until incorporated.

03. In a separate medium sized bowl, add flaxseed meal, buckwheat flour, coconut flour, almond flour, Himalayan salt, baking powder, baking soda, Choice Superfood Protein, and Pumpkin Spice and mix well.

04. Add the dry ingredients to the bowl with the wet ingredients and mix to combine. Pour batter into the lined loaf pan.

05. Bake for 30 minutes, or until a toothpick comes out clean. Edges should be slightly browned.

PUMPKIN SPICE

INGREDIENTS:

3 TBSP
Ground Cinnamon

4 TSP
Ground Ginger

½ TSP
Ground Nutmeg

¼ TSP
Ground Clove

⅛ TSP
Allspice

¼ TSP
Ground Black Pepper

¼ TSP
Ground Cardamom

PREPARATION:

01. Mix all ingredients together and use as you wish!

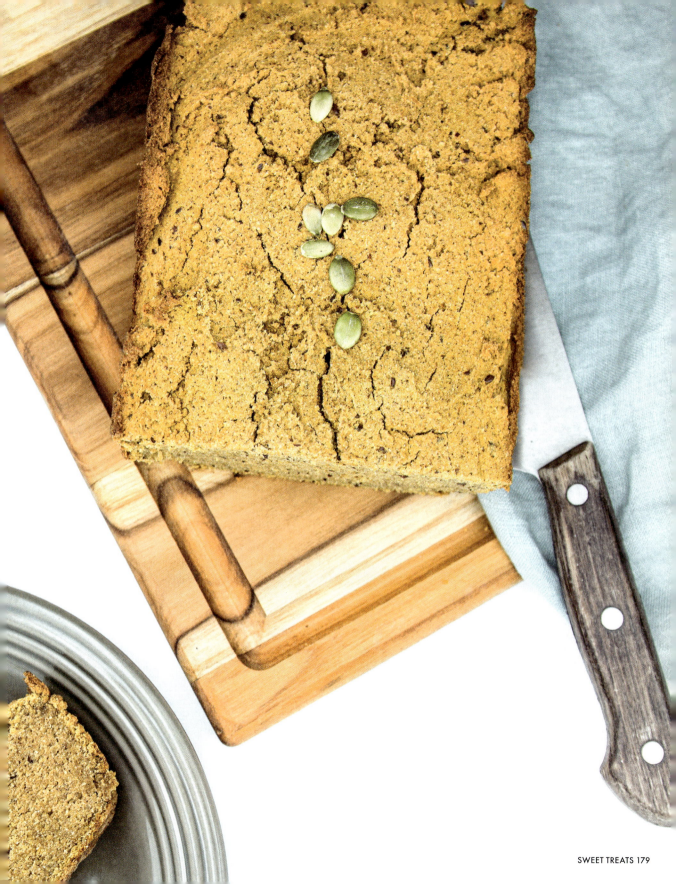

SWEET TREATS 179

PEANUT BUTTER CHICKPEA COOKIES

I love all things peanut butter, but traditional peanut butter cookies are often full of processed flours, unhealthy oils and way too much sugar. This is a healthier version of a traditional peanut butter cookie. It's time consuming to remove the chickpea skins, but absolutely necessary.

INGREDIENTS:

- 1/3 CUP Gluten-Free Rolled Oats
- 1/2 CUP Peanut Butter
- 1 CUP Canned Chickpeas, drained, rinsed, skins removed (important step)
- 1/2 CUP Agave
- 1/8 TSP Himalayan Salt
- 1/2 TSP Pure Vanilla Extract

PREPARATION:

01. Preheat the oven to 350°F.

02. In a food processor, blend oats until a fine "oat flour" texture is achieved. Add remaining ingredients to the food processor and blend until smooth.

03. Portion dough into 12 balls, and place onto a parchment lined sheet tray. Gently flatten balls by pressing down with fork twice, making the classic Peanut Butter Cookie design on each round.

04. Bake for 15 minutes (or until slightly golden). Let cool for 10 minutes on a cooling rack before serving (unless you like them warm like I do - yum!).

GUILT FREE CHOCOLATE CHIP COOKIES

INGREDIENTS:

- 3/4 CUP Oat Flour
- 1 15OZ. CAN Chickpeas, rinsed and drained and peeled.
- 3/4 CUP Coconut Sugar
- 3 TBSP Coconut Oil, melted
- 1 TBSP Pure Vanilla Extract
- 1/2 TSP Himalayan Salt
- 1/2 TSP Baking Soda
- 1 TSP Apple Cider Vinegar
- 1/2 CUP Vegan Chocolate Chips (more if you like them extra chocolatey)

PREPARATION:

01. Preheat the oven to 350°F.

02. In a medium sized bowl, combine the oat flour, baking soda, and Himalayan salt and set aside.

03. In a Vitamix or food processor, blend the chickpeas, coconut sugar, coconut oil, vanilla, and apple cider vinegar until smooth.

04. Add the smooth chickpea mixture to the dry ingredients and work together until well combined. Fold in the chocolate chips and spoon onto lightly greased cookie sheet, or a parchment paper lined sheet pan.

05. Bake for 15 minutes (checking towards the end of the cooking process to make sure they don't burn on the bottom). These cookies will be soft and gooey, and will blow your mind when you realize you're eating garbanzo beans!

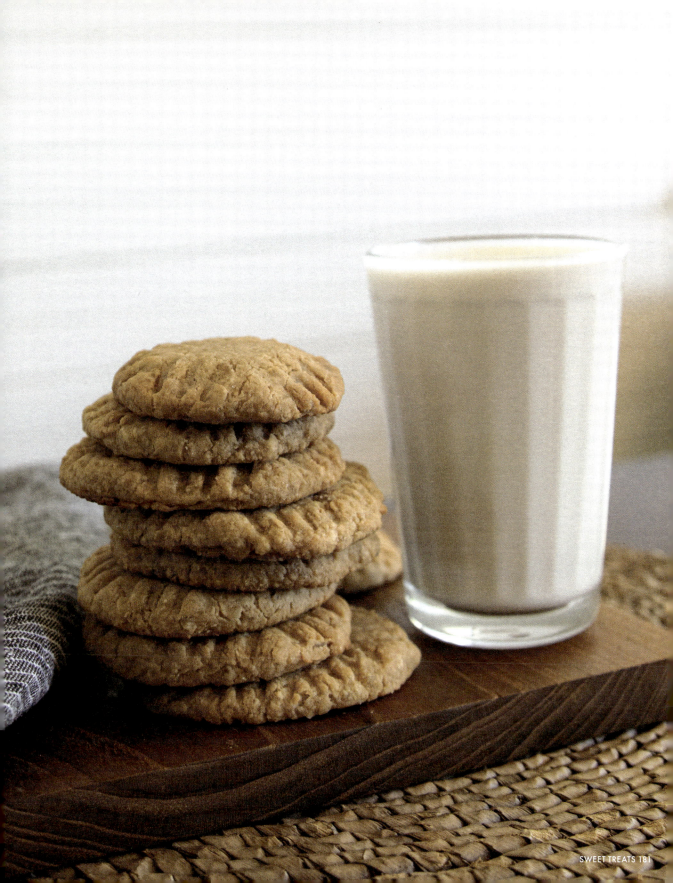

CHOCOLATE AVOCADO MOUSSE

We made this one year for our company holiday party and we've been hooked ever since. By popular demand, this dish now makes an appearance at all of our company gatherings. It's a sinfully rich, ultra silky Chocolate Avocado Mousse that will blow your mind!

INGREDIENTS:

3 LARGE
Avocados

3/4 CUP
Cacao Powder

4-5 TBSP
Sprouted Vanilla Almond Milk

1/4 TSP
Himalayan Salt

1/2 CUP
Pure Maple Syrup

3/4 TSP
Pure Vanilla Extract

PREPARATION:

01. Add all ingredients to a blender and blend until completely smooth.

02. Pour into a serving dish or 3 dessert ramekins, and refrigerate until firm (about 2 hours).

03. Serve on it's own, or top with cacao nibs, fresh berries, coconut whipped cream and coconut caramel (SEE RECIPE ON PG. 210)

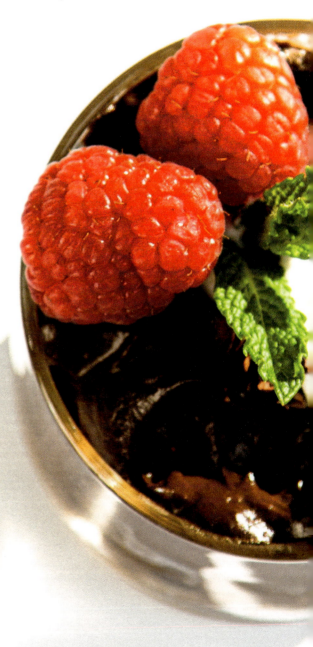

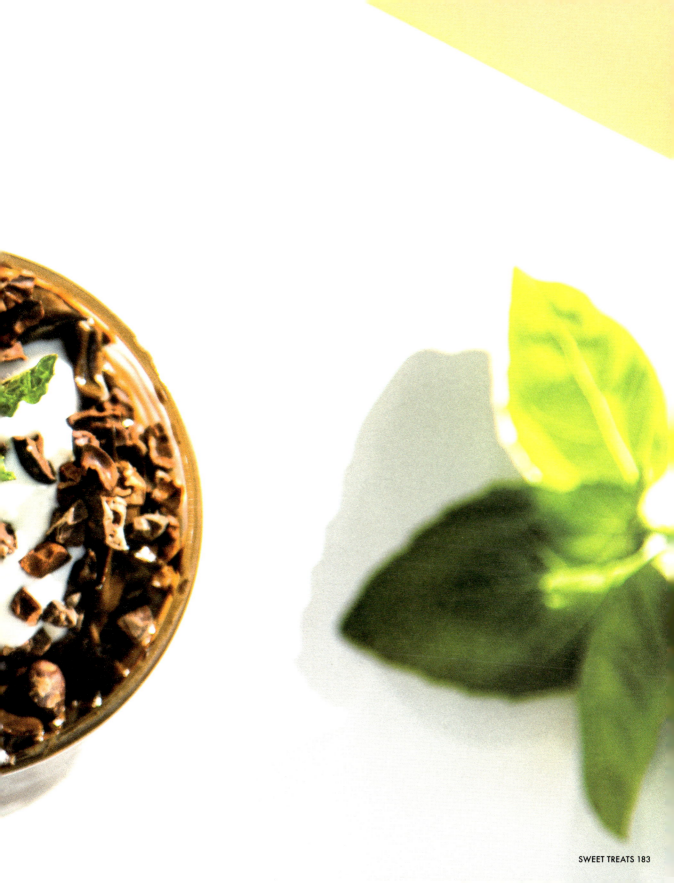

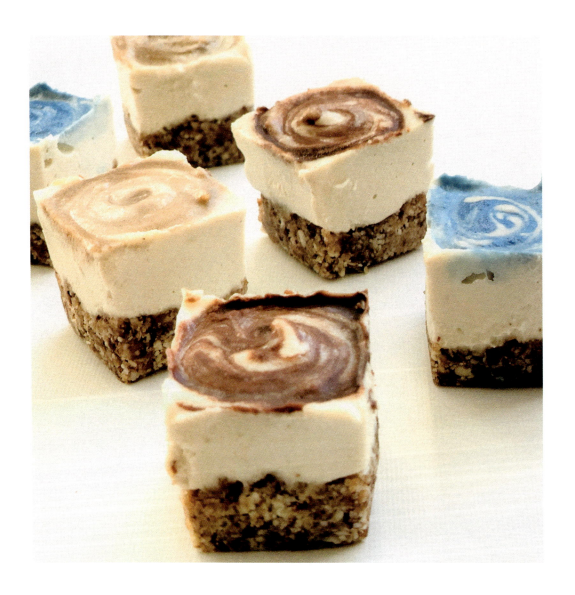

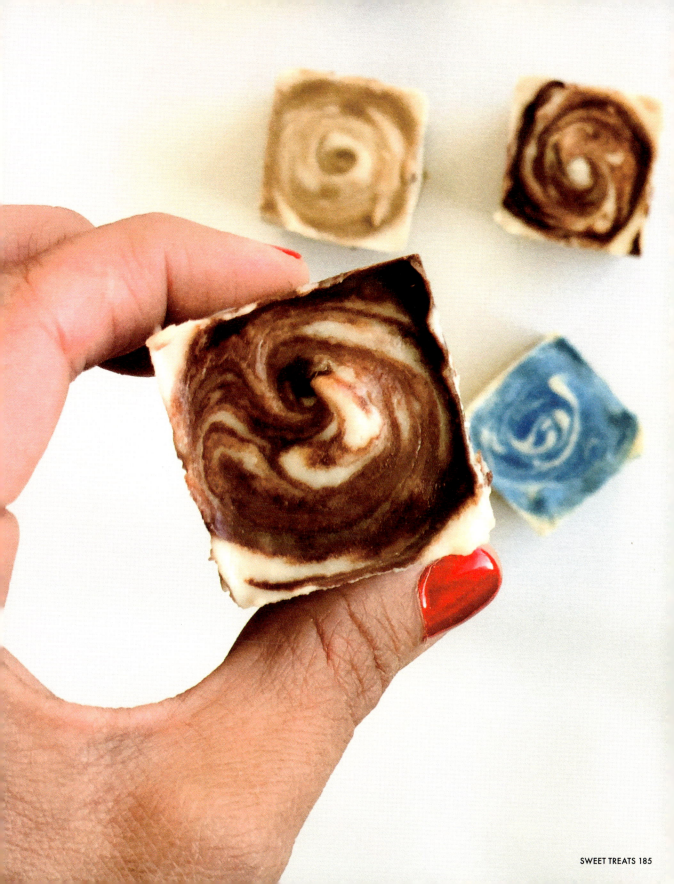

CHEESECAKE BITES

These cheesecake bites are easy to make, super yummy and filled with nutrition. What more could you ask for out of a sweet treat? And yes, they're vegan too.

ALMOND CRUST
INGREDIENTS:

½ CUP
Raw Almonds

½ CUP
Shredded Coconut

8 LARGE
Medjool Dates, pitted

⅛ TSP
Himalayan Salt

FOR CHEESECAKE

2 CUPS
Raw Cashews, soaked for at least 2 hours

½ CUP
Coconut Milk
NOTE:
You can use homemade Coconut Milk (SEE RECIPE ON PG. 50) or a canned coconut milk. If you opt for canned coconut milk, scoop out and use the solidified coconut cream that forms on the top.

½ CUP + 2 TBSP
Pure Maple Syrup

⅓ CUP
Coconut Oil, melted

¼ CUP
Lemon Juice

1 ½ TSP
Pure Vanilla Extract

PINCH
Himalayan Salt

NOTE:
I love to make these cheesecake bites in mini cupcake pans, or little square molds. If you choose to make these in cupcake pans, lining the cups with strips of parchment paper (or cupcake wrappers) makes removal super easy. You can also use a square baking dish or a small springform pan and portion the cheesecake into bite-sized pieces after it sets.

CRUST
PREPARATION:

01. Place all ingredients into a food processor and pulse until a crumbly texture is achieved. Over blending can turn this Almond Crust into an almond butter, so take care to not over blend.

02. When the Almond Crust is blended, spread the mixture onto the bottom of the molds, pressing into the pan to form a crust.

CHEESECAKE

01. Mix all of the ingredients in a high powered blender. I know it is a bummer to have to use and clean both a blender and food processor, but you want to use the blender on this step to really get the creamy texture you're looking for!

02. For Blue Majik swirled cheesecake bites, set aside ¼ of the cheesecake batter before pouring. Otherwise, pour the cheesecake batter over the Almond Crust. At this stage, these Cheesecake Bites can be enhanced by swirling in one of the 3 Cheesecake Toppings...totally optional, and totally unforgettable!

03. Place your cheesecake into the freezer to set for *at least an hour*. Remove cheesecake from the freezer 30 minutes before serving. It should be firm. The longer it sits out, the less firm it will become, so timing is key!

NOTE:
Can be kept in the freezer for up to 2 weeks.

3 CHEESECAKE TOPPING OPTIONS

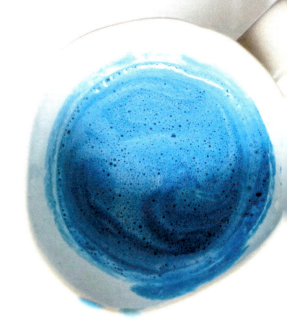

CHOCOLATE SAUCE SWIRL
INGREDIENTS:

½ CUP
Water

2 TBSP
Pure Maple Syrup or Monk Fruit
(+ more to taste)

½ CUP
Cacao Powder

2 TBSP
Cacao Butter, chopped

1 PINCH
Himalayan Salt

1 TSP
Pure Vanilla Extract

COCONUT CARAMEL SAUCE
(SEE RECIPE ON PG. 210)

CHOCOLATE SAUCE SWIRL
PREPARATION:

01. Heat all ingredients in a small saucepan until cacao butter is melted and Chocolate Sauce is smooth.

02. Place a dollop of chocolate sauce on top of the top of the cheesecake bites and swirl into the filling with a toothpick

BLUE MAJIK SWIRL

01. Take ¼ cup cheesecake filling and mix with 1 tsp E3Live Blue Majik

02. Place a dollop of blue cheesecake filling on top of the top of the cheesecake bites and swirl into the filling with a toothpick.

COCONUT CARAMEL SWIRL

01. Place a dollop of Coconut Caramel Sauce on top of the top of the cheesecake bites and swirl into the filling with a toothpick

RAW CHOCOLATE TRUFFLES

This is a great way to put your almond pulp to use and satisfy your sweet tooth at the same time. These rich, sweet, chocolatey truffles contain protein and maca, keeping you fueled and feeling energized! They're a great post or pre-workout treat!

INGREDIENTS:

HEAPING 1/2 CUP
Almond Pulp (SEE NOTE)

1/3 CUP
Almond Butter

6 LARGE
Medjool Dates, pitted

3 1/2 TBSP
Cacao Powder

1 1/2 TSP
Maca Powder

1/4 TSP
Himalayan Salt (+ more to taste)

COATING OPTIONS:

COCONUT SHREDS

HEMP SEEDS

CACAO NIBS

PREPARATION:

01. Add almond pulp, almond butter, medjool dates, cacao, maca and salt to a food processor. Process until dough like consistency is formed.

02. Portion into 12 balls, and roll in your choice of coatings (listed above). I like to do a combo of all three.

03. These are ready to enjoy or can be stored in an airtight container in the refrigerator for up to 5 days.

NOTE:
Almond pulp is the by-product of almond milk. If you don't have any almond pulp on hand, you can substitute almond flour. When using almond flour in place of almond pulp, increase the almond butter in the recipe by 2 - 4 Tbsp.

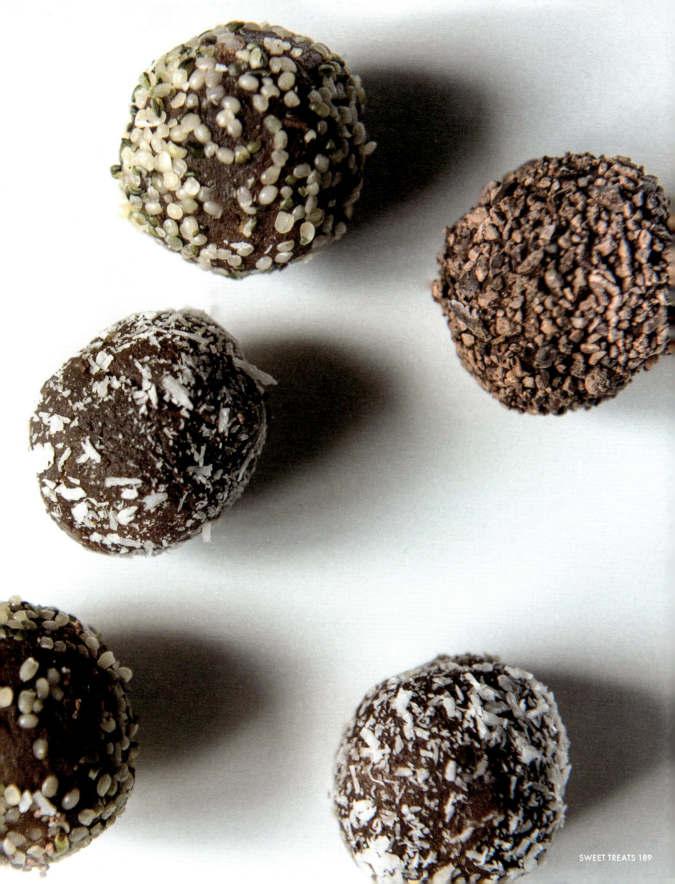

CHAPTER 15

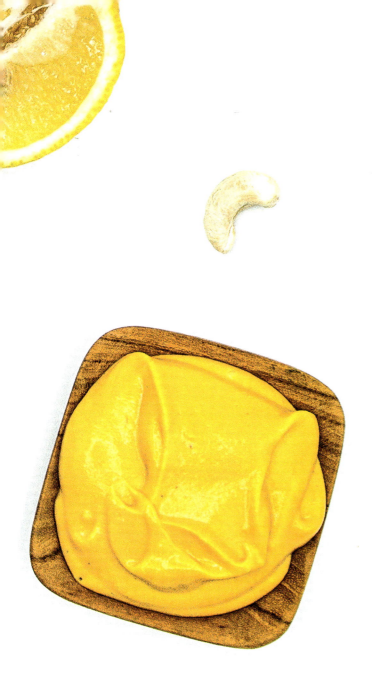

SAUCES, DRESSINGS & TOPPINGS

I love sauces! So if you're anything like me, then you will love this chapter, which is a collection of some of my favorite saucy recipes. While the recipes in this section go with the recipes throughout this book, they can be used in so many different ways. Have fun experimenting! The "cheese" sauces are incredible in burritos, enchiladas, nachos and mac n' "cheese." The sauces can be used as dips, dressings or on top of your own fun creations. I'm certain adding these recipes to your repertoire will take your vegan cooking to the next level.

MAC 'N "CHEESE" SAUCE

This is my favorite Mac 'N "Cheese" sauce, hands down! My kids absolutely love it, and I love that it's made with veggies. This sauce is a staple in our home, and it's not just for mac 'n "cheese"! It's awesome in other pasta dishes, enchiladas, on top of Buddha bowls... the possibilities are endless!

INGREDIENTS:

1 CUP
Potatoes, peeled and diced

1/4 CUP
Carrot, peeled and diced

1/3 LARGE
White Onion, chopped

1 CLOVE
Garlic

3/4 CUPS
Water (reserve from boiled vegetables)

1/2 CUP
Raw Cashews, soaked overnight (or minimum of 1 hour in hot water)

2 TBSP
Nutritional Yeast

1 TBSP
Lemon Juice

1 TSP
Himalayan Salt (+ more to taste)

1/2 TSP
Garlic Powder

1/2 TSP
Onion Powder

PREPARATION:

01. Boil potatoes, carrot and onion and until soft. Strain (reserving 3/4 cups water for sauce + more to thin if necessary).

02. Add boiled vegetables, raw garlic, spices, cashews, lemon juice, and the reserved water from cooked veggies to a high powered blender and blend on high for 3 minutes. Taste and adjust salt and seasonings as needed.

CHIPOTLE "CHEESE" SAUCE

This sauce is always a crowd pleaser. I use this over enchiladas, in my burritos, on top of my lettuce wraps, as a dip, and of course, in some of the delicious recipes throughout this book.

INGREDIENTS:

1 CUP
Raw Cashews, soaked overnight (or minimum of 1 hour in hot water), drained and rinsed

1 LARGE
Chipotle Pepper in Adobo sauce (+ more to taste, depending on how spicy you like your sauce. Chipotle in Adobo Sauce is usually found in the Mexican food isle and in a small can)

3 TBSP
Lemon Juice

1/2 TSP
Himalayan Salt (+ more to taste)

1 CLOVE
Garlic

3 TBSP
Nutritional Yeast

2 TSP
Pure Maple Syrup

1/2 CUP
Water (+ more to thin sauce, as needed)

PREPARATION:

01. Add all ingredients to a high powered blender and blend on high for 3 minutes, or until sauce is smooth. Add extra water until desired consistency is achieved. Adjust seasonings accordingly, and taste as you go!

NACHO "CHEESE" SAUCE

This Nacho "Cheese" Sauce is absolutely crave-worthy! It has a smooth and creamy texture, and a great depth of flavor that goes well with everything from tacos to roasted veggies. The jalapeño adds just the right amount of spice, you'll find yourself enjoying this "cheese" on top of more than just nachos!

<u>NOTE</u>:
Jalapeños vary in spice. It's always a safe bet to test your jalapeño beforehand to see what you are working with. If you lucked out and got a super spicy one, add half of what the recipe calls for to start and taste before adding more. You can always add more, but you can never remove after the fact.

INGREDIENTS:

1 CUP
Potatoes, peeled and diced

1/4 CUP
Carrot, peeled and diced

1/3
White Onion, chopped

1 CLOVE
Garlic

3/4 CUPS
Water (reserve from boiled vegetables)

2 TBSP
Nutritional Yeast

1 TBSP
Lemon Juice

1 TSP
Himalayan Salt
(+ more to taste)

1/2 TSP
Garlic Powder

1/2 TSP
Onion Powder

1/2 CUP
Raw Cashews, soaked overnight (or minimum of 1 hour in hot water)

1/4 CUP
Red Bell Pepper, diced

1/2
Jalapeño, seeded and minced

1/4 TSP
Paprika

PREPARATION:

01. Boil potatoes, carrot and onion until soft. Strain (reserving ¾ cups water for sauce + more to thin if necessary).

02. Add all remaining ingredients to a high powered blender and blend on high for 3 minutes. Taste and adjust salt and seasonings as needed.

LEMON GARLIC TAHINI DRESSING

Tahini is an incredible superfood. It's essentially a nut butter made from sesame seeds, but that's where the similarities end. The list of health benefits goes on and on. Tahini is loaded with magnesium, phosphorus, calcium, iron and potassium. It's full of healthy fats and omega-3s that may lower cholesterol and fight inflammation, and tahini contains more protein than milk and most nuts.

Studies show raw tahini may improve skin health, heart health, and bone health. It's a rich source of B vitamins that boost energy and brain function. Plus, tahini contains vitamin E, which is protective against heart disease and stroke. Eating tahini regularly can help prevent iron deficiency, which leads to fatigue and low blood cell count. It's also full of copper, zinc, and selenium. So, it's essentially an immune system savior.

The more you read about it, the more it sounds like a miracle food. And in my humble opinion, it really is!

INGREDIENTS:

1/2 CUP
Raw Tahini

1/4 - 1/2 CUP
Water (add ¼ to start and add additional water as needed to thin out dressing)

6 TBSP
Lemon Juice

1/2 TSP
Himalayan Salt
(+ more to taste)

1/2 TSP
Onion Powder

2 CLOVES
Garlic

1 TBSP
Agave

PREPARATION:

01. Add all ingredients to a blender and blend on high for 1-2 minutes, until smooth. Can be stored in an airtight container for up to 5 days.

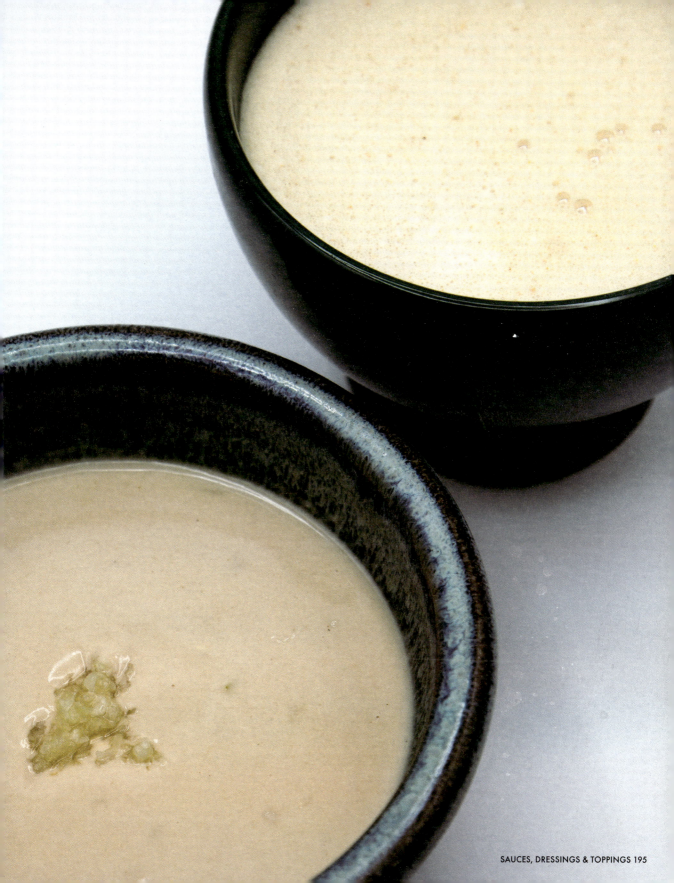

SAUCES, DRESSINGS & TOPPINGS 195

CAESAR DRESSING

(MAKES 2 CUPS; CAN BE STORED UP TO 6 DAYS IN FRIDGE)

INGREDIENTS:

3/4 CUP
Raw Cashews, soaked overnight (or minimum of 1 hour in hot water), drained and rinsed.

1/2 CUP
Water

3 TBSP
Olive Oil

1 CLOVE
Garlic

1 1/2 TBSP
Lemon Juice

1 1/2 TBSP
Capers

2 1/2 TSP
Mustard

2 1/2 TSP
Vegan Worcestershire

3/4 TSP
Garlic Powder

3/4 TSP
Himalayan Salt

3/4 TSP
Black Pepper

PREPARATION:

01. Combine all ingredients in a high powered blender, and blend until very smooth (about 4 minutes).

"SOUR CREAM" & ONION DRESSING

INGREDIENTS:

1 CUP
Raw Cashews, soaked in hot water for 35 minutes

2/3 CUP
Water (+ more to thin)

2 TBSP
Onion Powder

1/2 TSP
Garlic Powder

2 TBSP
Lemon Juice

1 1/2 TSP
Apple Cider Vinegar

1/2 TSP
Himalayan Salt (+ more to taste)

1/4 CUP
Fresh Parsley, minced

2 TBSP
Nutritional Yeast

PREPARATION:

01. Blend all ingredients in a high powered blender for 60 seconds until smooth.

CASHEW RANCH DRESSING

People constantly ask if they can buy the Cashew Ranch Dressing at Choice. It's dresses one of our signature salads, the Coconut "Bakon" Cobb. The truth is, this Cashew Ranch Dressing is so good, you'll want to use it for more than just salads! It's rich in potassium, iron, magnesium, manganese, calcium, vitamin A, K, C and protein. So many reasons to eat this unbelievably delicious dressing on everything!

INGREDIENTS:
(1ST SET)

1 CUP
Raw Cashews, soaked

3/4 CUP
Water

1 1/2 TBSP
Lemon Juice

1 1/2 TBSP
Apple Cider Vinegar

1 1/2 TBSP
Garlic Powder

1 1/2 TBSP
Onion Powder

1 TSP
Himalayan Salt

2 TSP
Black Pepper

(2ND SET)

1/2 TSP
Dried Dill

1 TSP
Fresh Parsley, chopped

3 TBSP
Olive Oil

PREPARATION:

01. Soak cashews in cold water for at least 2 hours, or up to overnight. Cashews can also be soaked in hot water for 30 minutes.

02. Add the ingredients from the first set to a high powered blender and blend on high for 1-2 minutes, or until dressing is smooth.

03. Add dill and parsley from the second set of ingredients to the blender and blend for about 10 seconds. Slowly stream in the olive oil.

"ALFREDO" SAUCE

This "Alfredo" sauce is high in protein, fiber and minerals. It's also immune boosting, energizing, metabolism boosting, alkalizing and it contains iron and omega-3s. Oh and it happens to be one of the best tasting "Alfredo" sauces you'll ever have!

INGREDIENTS:

1 ½ CUPS
Raw Cashews, soaked

1 ¼ CUPS
Water

3 CLOVES
Garlic

1 TBSP
Lemon Juice

1 ½ TSP
Onion Powder

3 TBSP
Nutritional Yeast

1 ½ TSP
Himalayan Salt

⅓ TSP
Rosemary

PREPARATION:

01. Soak cashews in cold water for at least 2 hours, or up to overnight. Cashews can also be soaked in hot water for 30 minutes.

02. Add all ingredients to a blender and blend until very smooth (about 1 minute).

03. Use immediately.

NOTE:

The "Alfredo" sauce may be slightly warm from blending, and can be further heated on the stove top over low flame. Otherwise, pour into a sealed container and store for up to 5 days.

BBQ SAUCE (MAKES 4 CUPS: CAN BE STORED UP TO 2 WEEKS)

This BBQ Sauce is healthy, spicy, rich, slightly smokey, and super easy to make!

INGREDIENTS:

1 1/2 CUPS
Sun Dried Tomatoes

2 3/4 CUPS
Water

3/4 CUP
Agave

1 1/2 TSP
Gluten-Free Tamari

1 1/2 TSP
Rice Wine Vinegar

1 1/2 TSP
Apple Cider Vinegar

1 1/2 TSP
Dried Oregano

1/2 TSP
Garlic Powder

1/2 TSP
Onion Powder

2 TSP
Chipotle Powder

2 1/2 TSP
Black Pepper

2/3 TSP
Paprika

1 TSP
Vegan Worcestershire

1 TSP
Liquid Smoke

PREPARATION:

01. Add all ingredients to a high powered blender and blend on high until smooth.

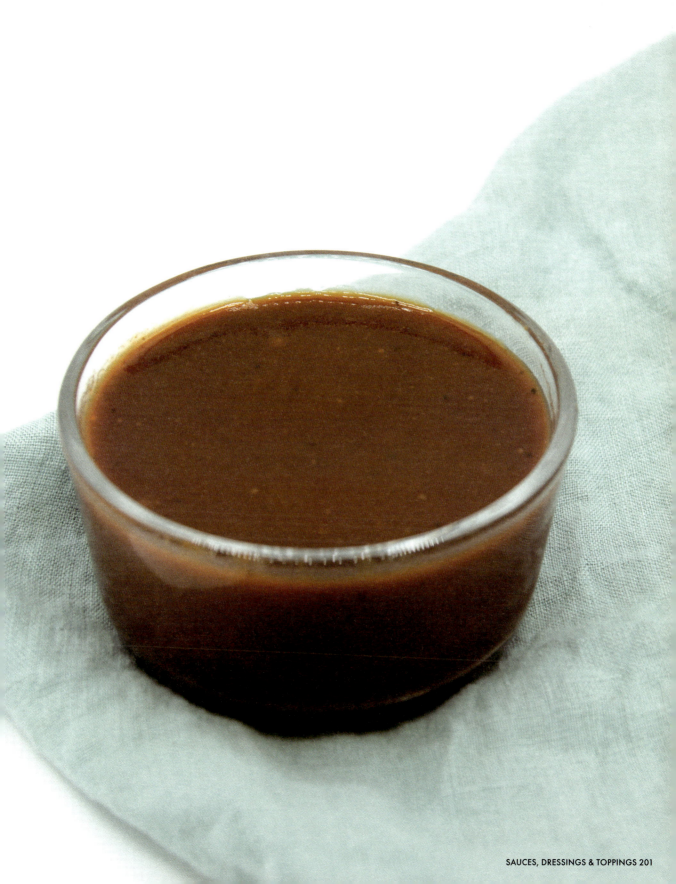

SUN DRIED TOMATO PESTO

This is a fun spin on a traditional pesto. I love sun dried tomatoes! In the summer, I always end up with more tomatoes than I know what to do with from my garden. So naturally, I make sun dried tomatoes because they're delicious. I'm always looking for fun ways to use my sun dried tomatoes and this recipe was a win for me and my kiddos.

INGREDIENTS:
(MAKES ABOUT 1 ¾ CUPS)

1 CUP
Sun Dried Tomatoes, packed in oil (drained)

1 CUP
Pine Nuts, roasted (in a dry pan on low heat for 5 minutes)

¼ CUP
Fresh Basil, packed

3 TBSP
Olive Oil (+ more as needed)

3 TBSP
Lemon Juice

½ CUPS
Water (start with ¼ and add to thin)

⅓ CUP
Nutritional Yeast

½ TSP
Himalayan Salt

¼ TSP
Black Pepper

3 CLOVES
Garlic

PREPARATION:

01. Place all ingredients in a food processor and process until you have pesto!

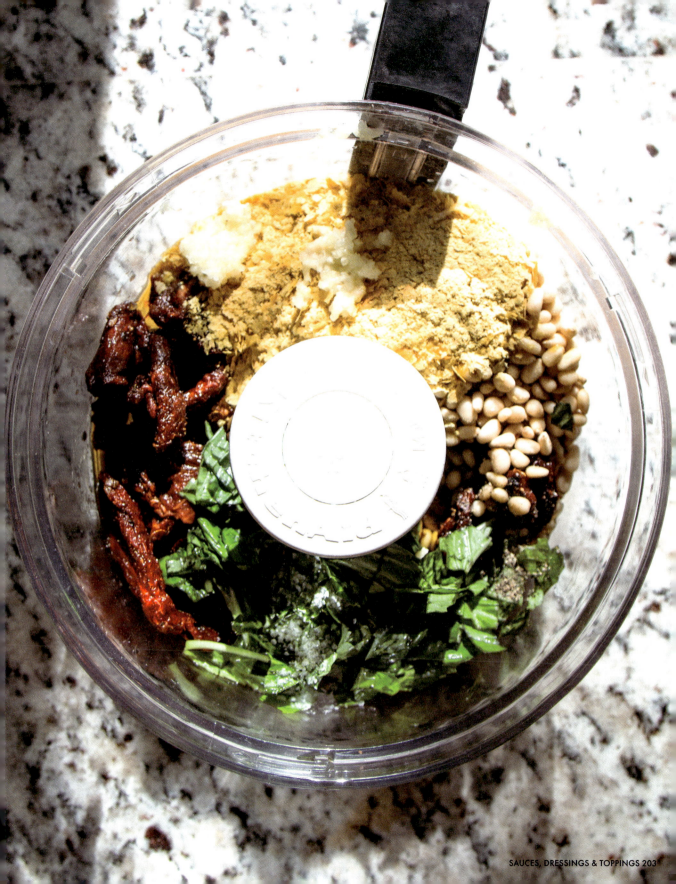

MISO GINGER SAUCE

INGREDIENTS:

1 ¼ CUP
Ginger, peeled and chopped

2 CLOVES
Garlic

2 TBSP
Chickpea Miso
(SEE NOTE)

2 TBSP
Rice Wine Vinegar

1 TBSP
Tahini

¼ CUP
Water
(+ more to thin, as needed)

1 TBSP
Agave

2 TBSP
Lemon Juice

1 TBSP
Sesame Oil

PREPARATION:

01. Place ingredients (except sesame oil) into a high powered blender and blend until smooth, about 2 minutes

02. Once desired consistency is achieved, slowly stream in sesame oil to emulsify.

03. Fresh ginger can be fibrous. For a smooth sauce, strain through a fine sieve.

NOTE:
If your health food store doesn't carry chickpea miso, mellow white miso or light yellow miso can be substituted.

PAD THAI SAUCE

Who doesn't love a good Pad Thai sauce? I am a huge fan of Thai Cuisine. I'm always looking for ways to healthify and veganize my favorite dishes and sauces, and this sauce does just that! Healthy, vegan, and Thai inspired, it's a great dipping sauce and is divine on Kelp Noodle Pad Thai (SEE RECIPE ON PG. 162).

INGREDIENTS:

1/4 CUP Lemon Juice

2 TSP Ginger, grated

1 CLOVE Garlic

1 TBSP Gluten-Free Tamari

1/2 CUP Peanut Butter

1 TBSP Cilantro, packed

1 TBSP Basil, packed

1/2 Jalapeño, seeded

1/4 TSP Toasted Sesame Oil

3/4 CUPS Water (+ more to thin, as needed)

1 TSP Himalayan Salt

1 TBSP Agave

1 TSP Rice Wine Vinegar

PREPARATION:

01. Place all ingredients in a high powered blender and blend until smooth and creamy, about 2 minutes.

SPICY CASHEW AIOLI

INGREDIENTS:

1 CUP Raw Cashews, soaked

1/2 CUP Water (+ more to thin)

2 1/2 TBSP Lemon Juice

1 CLOVE Garlic

2 TBSP Nutritional Yeast

2 TSP Organic Sriracha Chili Sauce, + more to taste (or use your favorite organic chili sauce)

1/4 TSP Garlic Powder

1/4 TSP Onion Powder

1/2 TSP Himalayan Salt (or to taste)

PREPARATION:

01. Place all ingredients in a high powered blender and blend on high for 2 minutes, stopping to add more water, as needed.

02. Once the Spicy Cashew Aioli is smooth, transfer to an airtight container and store in the refrigerator for up to 5 days.

NOTE:

I love my vitamix, but if you don't have one, make sure your cashews are soaked well so they blend smoothly.

COCONUT "BAKON"

Sometimes you just need that smokey taste to finish off a recipe. These Coconut "Bakon" flakes are the perfect addition to your salads, soups, or even a homemade CBLT sammy (coconut "bakon", lettuce, tomato - on gluten-free bread of course).

INGREDIENTS:

2 TBSP
Liquid Smoke

2 TBSP
Gluten-Free Tamari

2 TBSP
Pure Maple Syrup

½ TBSP
Coconut Oil, melted

1 ½ TSP
Water

2 CUPS
Large Coconut Flakes
(not shreds)

DASH
Himalayan Salt and Pepper

PREPARATION:

01. Preheat the oven to 275°F.

02. In a medium sized bowl, whisk together liquid smoke, gluten-free tamari, pure maple syrup, coconut oil, water, salt and pepper.

03. Add coconut flakes to the bowl, gently tossing together. Let the coconut marinate for 10 minutes.

04. Prepare a baking sheet with oil. Spread marinated coconut on a baking sheet.

05. Bake at 275°F for 15-18 minutes, flipping every 5 minutes (important step as it burns easily).

06. Remove Coconut "Bakon" from the oven when it's nicely browned and mostly dry. The "Bakon" will crisp as it cools. Store at room temperature in an airtight container for up to 2 weeks, or up to a month in the freezer.

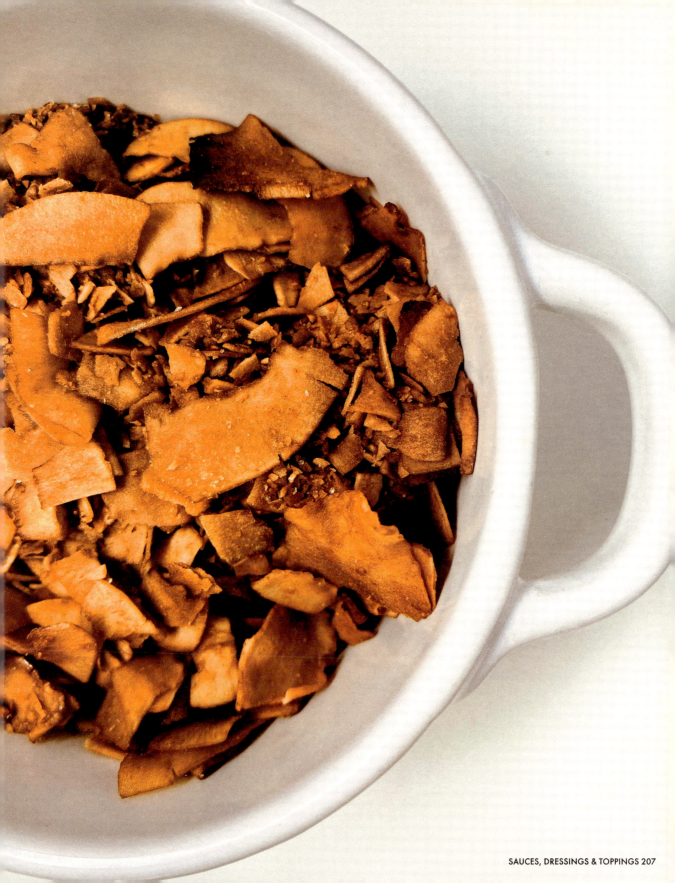

BRAZIL NUT "PARMESAN"

INGREDIENTS:

½ CUP
Raw Brazil Nuts

3 TBSP
Raw Cashews

3 TBSP
Hemp Seeds

3 TBSP
Nutritional Yeast

1 ½ TSP
Himalayan Salt

¾ TSP
Garlic Powder

PREPARATION:

01. Combine Brazil nuts, cashews and hemp seeds in a blender or food processor. Pulse until a sandy texture is achieved. Be careful! Pulsing too much can result in a Brazil nut butter!

02. Add the remaining ingredients into the blender and pulse again until you have a "parmesan" consistency. Again, be careful not to over blend.

03. Store in an airtight container for up to 2 weeks.

VEGAN SLAW

INGREDIENTS:

2 CUPS
Carrots, shredded

2 CUPS
Purple Cabbage, shredded

2 CUPS
Green Cabbage, shredded
(or 4 cups of whatever cabbage you have on hand)

1 CUP
Raw Cashews (soaked in hot water for a minimum of 1 hour, or overnight in cold water and then rinsed and drained.

1 ½ TBSP
Pure Maple Syrup or Agave

⅓ CUP
Water

1 TBSP
Spicy Mustard

2 TBSP
White Vinegar

1 TBSP
Apple Cider Vinegar

3 TBSP
Yellow Onion, chopped

½ TSP
Celery Salt

Himalayan Salt & Black Pepper, to taste

PREPARATION:

01. Combine cabbage and carrots in a large bowl and set aside.

02. Blend all slaw dressing ingredients in a high speed blender until smooth. Taste and adjust as necessary.

03. Add the dressing to your cabbage carrot slaw and toss to coat the veggies evenly. You can use this immediately or you can place it in the fridge to chill. If you prefer to make it in advance, you can cover it and leave it in the fridge for roughly 5 days.

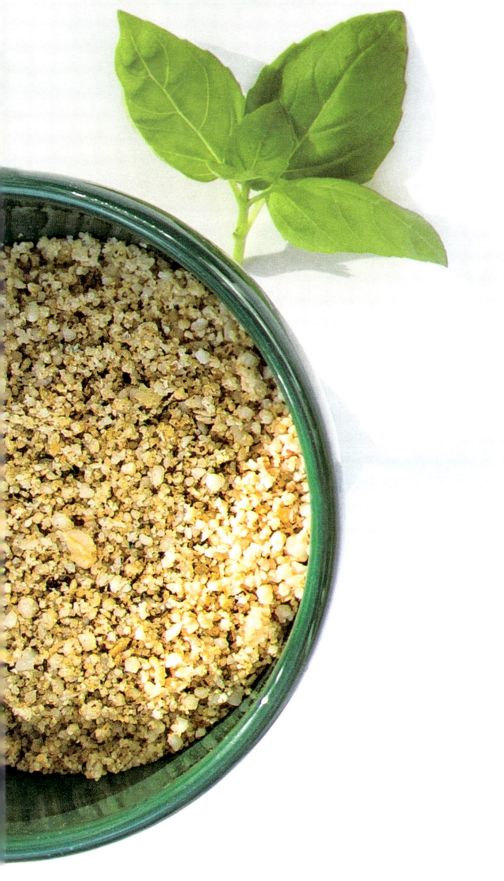

COCONUT WHIPPED CREAM

Decadent, fluffy, plant-based whipped cream can easily be made by using a can of full-fat coconut milk. Not only is the technique simple, but I think it's the best tasting "whipped cream" EVER! You can use this Coconut Whipped Cream just like regular dairy whipped cream. I like to use it on top of my lattés, over a Chocolate Avocado Mousse, with some fresh berries or on top of a slice of pie. The options are endless!

INGREDIENTS:

1 14 OZ. CAN
Full-Fat Coconut Milk, chilled for 24 hours *(SEE NOTE)* - It's important that the coconut milk is full fat, and free of guar gum. Check the ingredients!

2 TBSP
Pure Maple Syrup or Agave

½ TSP
Pure Vanilla Extract

NOTE:
Place the can of full-fat coconut milk in the refrigerator overnight. This is a crucial step. The coconut cream needs to be chilled until very firm, otherwise it will not whip.

PREPARATION:

01. Before beginning, place a medium sized mixing bowl in the freezer for a few minutes. This helps keep everything cold. Remove the chilled can of coconut milk from the refrigerator and flip it upside down. The liquid coconut milk (the part that doesn't harden) will now be at the top of the can! Note: works with most cans of coconut milk!

02. Open the can of coconut milk and drain the liquid for later use (think smoothies, or soup!).

03. Scoop the solidified coconut cream into the chilled bowl and add pure maple syrup or agave, and vanilla.

04. Grab a hand mixer or a whisk and whip the ingredients until light and fluffy. Use immediately!

NOTE:
This Coconut Whipped Cream can be made in advance and stored in the refrigerator, but may need to be re-whipped before use.

COCONUT CARAMEL SAUCE (MAKES 1 CUP)

Use this decadent Coconut Caramel Sauce to top smoothie bowls, swirl into Cheesecake Bites, drizzle over desserts, or anything else your heart can dream up!

INGREDIENTS:

2 TBSP
Pure Maple Syrup

¼ CUP
Coconut Sugar

¼ CUP
Water

2 TBSP
Raw Cashews (do not soak)

2 LARGE
Medjool Dates, pitted

½ TSP
Pure Vanilla Extract

PINCH
Himalayan Salt

2 TBSP
Coconut Oil (do not melt)

NOTE:
Store this in the refrigerator for up to a week, and stir before using.

PREPARATION:

01. Add all ingredients (except coconut oil) into a vitamix and blend until very smooth.

02. Add coconut oil last and blend until combined.

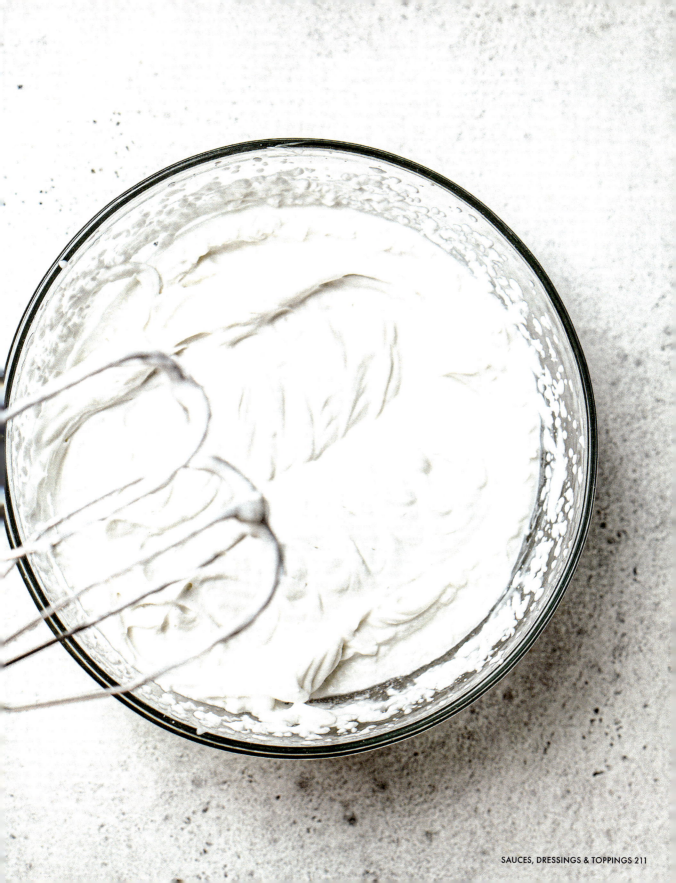

RESOURCE PAGE

CHAPTER 1
https://www.pcrm.org/good-nutrition/plant-based-diets
https://www.cowspiracy.com/facts
https://www.whatthehealthfilm.com/facts
https://www.dosomething.org/us/facts/11-facts-about-animals-and-factory-farms
https://www.onegreenplanet.org/animalsandnature/facts-about-the-lives-of-factory-farmed-animals/
https://www.whatthehealthfilm.com/facts
https://www.cowspiracy.com
https://www.dosomething.org/us/facts/11-facts-about-animals-and-factory-farms
https://www.onegreenplanet.org/animalsandnature/facts-about-the-lives-of-factory-farmed-animals/
https://www.dosomething.org/us/facts/11-facts-about-animals-and-factory-farms

CHAPTER 2
https://www.huffingtonpost.ca/2013/07/25/camu-camu-benefits-_n_3644392.html
https://www.huffingtonpost.ca/2013/07/25/camu-camu-benefits-_n_3644392.html
https://www.foodmatters.com/article/powerful-health-benefits-of-acai-berry
https://www.e3live.com/p-7-blue-majik.aspx
https://yoursuper.com/pages/spirulina-health-benefits
https://www.verywellhealth.com/the-benefits-of-white-mulberry-88659

CHAPTER 3
https://www.healthline.com/nutrition/10-proven-benefits-of-kale#TOC_TITLE_HDR_3
https://www.medicalnewstoday.com/articles/270678#benefits
https://www.ncbi.nlm.nih.gov/pmc/articles/PMC6018397/

CHAPTER 4
https://www.pcrm.org/good-nutrition/nutrition-information/health-concerns-about-dairy
https://www.ncbi.nlm.nih.gov/pmc/articles/PMC5601385/
https://www.sciencetimes.com/articles/27287/20200914/examining-anticancer-properties-coconut-oils.htm
https://www.sciencetimes.com/articles/27287/20200914/examining-anticancer-properties-coconut-oils.htm

CHAPTER 5
https://thehealthychef.com/blogs/wellbeing/why-matcha-is-good-for-weight-loss
https://www.healthline.com/health/food-nutrition/monk-fruit-health-benefits#health-benefits

CHAPTER 9
https://foodrevolution.org/blog/how-to-fight-prevent-cancer-with-mushrooms/

CHAPTER 10
https://www.theguardian.com/lifeandstyle/2013/mar/23/good-for-you-tahini

CHAPTER 11
https://www.healthline.com/nutrition/white-beans-nutrition

If you are interested in learning more about veganism or living a plant-based lifestyle in general, here are a few documentaries I highly recommend:

- Cowspiracy (Netflix)
- What the Health (Netflix)
- Speciesism (Netflix)
- Forks Over Knives (Netflix)
- Earthlings (Youtube)
- Meet your Meat (Youtube)

Books:
- Eating Animals
- The China Study
- The Food Revolution
- Diet For A New America
- The Cheese Trap